Meniscal Transplantation

René Verdonk · João Espregueira-Mendes
Joan Carles Monllau
Editors

Meniscal Transplantation

Springer

Editors
René Verdonk
Department of Orthopaedic Surgery and Traumatology
Ghent University Hospital,
Ghent
Belgium

João Espregueira-Mendes
Clínica Espregueira-Mendes: F. C: Porto Stadium Sports Center
Porto
Portugal

ICVS/3B's-PT Government Associate Laboratory
Headquarters of the European Institute of Excellence on Tissue Engineering and Regenerative Medicine
Braga
Portugal

and

3B's Research Group-Biomaterials
Biodegradables and Biomimetics
University of Minho
Guimarães
Portugal

Joan Carles Monllau
Department of Orthopaedic Surgery
Hospital de la Sta Creu i Sant Pau
Barcelona
Spain

ISBN 978-3-642-38105-8 ISBN 978-3-642-38106-5 (eBook)
DOI 10.1007/978-3-642-38106-5
Springer Heidelberg New York Dordrecht London

Library of Congress Control Number: 2013937195

Printed on acid-free paper

Springer is part of Springer Science+Business Media (www.springer.com)

Foreword

ISAKOS has a long tradition of education. My mentor, Prof. Dr. Ejnar Eriksson from Stockhom Sweden, always taught me that repetition was the mother of education.

This book on meniscal allograft and replacement is a good example of this principle.

Now that knowledge on this cartilage body in the knee has increased and experience has grown it is time again to confront this with our daily practice.

Once upon a time our orthopedic knowledge spanned the whole locomotor system pathology and treatment availabilities. More recently most of us started to focus on target diseases, abnormalities, and trauma sometimes forgetting the whole picture.

This is what happened to knee surgeons focusing on ligaments, cartilage, and the meniscus separately.

Although this work is edged towards meniscal pathology and replacement with expert clinicians sharing their expertise and knowledge, the interested reader should keep in mind that meniscal knowledge needs to be framed in the knee joint as a whole.

It is my personal experience, which I share with many others, that all elements of the "knee" puzzle should be accounted for when getting into knee pathology, diagnosis, and treatment.

To restore knee "homeostasis" as superbly described by my friend Dr. Scott Dye, all factors need to be coinciding towards healing.

Hopefully this book, next to many others as supported by the ISAKOS educational drive, will be part of the optimizing clinical approach and treatment in our sports dedicated patients and individuals.

Let me acknowledge all authors of this educational book for their intense collaboration to finalize this project and Mrs. Chantal Tielemans for her great help in additional editing and layout.

R. Verdonk

Contents

Part III The Future

Part IV Conclusion

Part I
Meniscal Allografts

Meniscal Allograft

1

R. Verdonk and P. Verdonk

1.1 Introduction

The purpose of this book is to look into meniscal disorders and their treatment options.

However, those who do not look back on history are bound to make the same mistakes…

That is the reason why in this chapter on basic knowledge of the meniscus, the phylogeny and ontogeny are dealt with first.

'Keep the meniscus' is the slogan based on the natural history of this disc of soft tissue in the knee joint, erroneously considered by some to be a vestigial soft-tissue structure in a 'self-maintaining transmission system'.

These combined sets of asymmetrical components meet the biomechanical need for load transference between the thigh and the leg so well that they have essentially persisted with minimal change for a period of over 300 million years of vertebrate evolution.

The knee thus represents a truly remarkable design of evolutionary biology.

Limbs occur very early in the ontological development of the human embryo, as do menisci in the evolutionary history of the human knee. By the end of the embryological period the menisci have become further defined and by nine to ten weeks they have become completely separated from the articular chondral surfaces of the tibia and femur.

R. Verdonk (✉)
Department of Orthopaedics and Trauma, Ghent University Hospital, De Pintelaan 185, 9000 Ghent, Belgium
e-mail: Rene.verdonk@ugent.be

P. Verdonk
Dept Orthopaedics and Trauma, Monica Ziekenhuizen, 2000 Antwerpen, Belgium

R. Verdonk et al. (eds.), *Meniscal Transplantation*,
DOI: 10.1007/978-3-642-38106-5_1, © ISAKOS 2013

The menisci remain of critical importance to the normal function of the knee joint.

As the menisci are sometimes referred to as 'semilunar cartilages', even though they are crescentic when viewed from above, they are wedge-shaped in cross-section and are attached to the joint capsule at their convex peripheral rim, except for a portion of the lateral meniscus in the region of the popliteus tendon, and also to the tibia anteriorly and posteriorly by insertional ligaments. They thus partially cover the tibiofemoral joint surface.

The circumferential collagen fibres of the meniscal body continue into the anterior and posterior insertional ligaments, which attach to the subchondral bone of the tibia. The insertional ligaments have fibrocartilaginous transition zones that make the change in stiffness between ligament and bone tissue at the enthesis less sudden, therefore reducing the stress concentration in this unit and preventing failure. In addition, the anterior intermeniscal ligament, also known as the transverse geniculate ligament, connects the anterior fibres of the anterior horns of the medial and lateral menisci. This anatomical finding has been identified in almost 94 % of cases and may have a role in moving the menisci during tibial internal-external rotation.

Two ligaments joining the posterior horn of the lateral meniscus to the lateral side of the medial femoral condyle in the intercondylar notch, have also been identified. The anterior meniscofemoral ligament runs anterior to the posterior cruciate ligament, and is known as the ligament of Humphrey. The posterior meniscofemoral ligament runs posterior to the posterior cruciate ligament, and is known as the ligament of Wrisberg.

A review of the literature by Gupte et al. suggested that at least one meniscofemoral ligament was present in 93 % of knees, with a significantly higher prevalence in younger knees than in older ones.

Normal meniscal tissue is composed of 72 % water, 22 % collagen, 0.8 % glycosaminoglycans and 0.12 % DNA.

Histologically, the menisci are fibrocartilaginous structures and are primarily composed of an interlacing network of collagen fibres interposed with cells, with an extracellular matrix of proteoglycans and glycoproteins.

The fine orientation of the collagen fibres within the meniscus is directly related to the function of the meniscus. The principal orientation of the collagen fibres is circumferential, to withstand tension. Radially oriented collagen fibres are predominantly present in the mid-portion of the meniscus and also on the exposed surfaces. These radial fibres might act as 'ties' holding the circumferential fibres together.

The entire meniscus is vascularized at birth. An avascular area soon develops in the inner portion of the meniscus, and in the second decade, blood vessels are only present in the outer third. The degree of vascularity varies within each meniscus.

Reports on the innervation of the menisci are conflicting. Wilson et al. also showed penetration of neural tissue into the outer third of the meniscus. The presence of mechanoreceptors in the menisci suggests that the menisci may play a role in knee joint afferent nerve transmission.

The menisci are dynamic structures, and to effectively maintain an optimum load-bearing function over a moving, incongruent joint surface, they need to be able to move with movements of the femur and tibia, in order to maintain maximum congruency.

Recent technical advances in the field of radiographic imaging have allowed in vivo studies of the intact knee under load in all positions. Vedi et al. have described meniscal motion in the normal knee in both weightbearing and non-weightbearing conditions.

Biomechanical investigations have looked into material properties of meniscal tissue.

In the literature, attempts have been made to quantify the meniscal response. A discrepancy exists between experimental studies on the variation of the tensile modulus along the circumference of the tissue.

Fewer studies have investigated the compressive properties of meniscal tissue. Menisci appear to be 1000 times stiffer in tension than in compression. These characteristics render the tissue very deformable in compression, which means that it can conform to the variable geometry of the femoral condyles during knee flexion and extension.

It has been well established that the main role of the menisci within the knee joint is transmission of the joint force from the femur to the tibia. This mechanism of loadbearing occurs throughout the whole range of knee-joint flexion precisely because the menisci are mainly attached to the tibia by insertional ligaments at their mobile horns, allowing displacement in all directions. The lateral meniscus is more mobile than the medial meniscus.

The resistance of the menisci to compressive loads by increasing their circumference and developing hoop stresses explains the variable effect and frequency of the various types of meniscal tears.

The shock-absorbing capacity of the menisci has been demonstrated by studies measuring the vibrations in the proximal tibia resulting from gait. Shock absorption has been shown to be approximately 20 % lower in knees without menisci.

Regarding the role of the menisci as secondary stabilizers within the knee, the clinical results of anterior cruciate ligament reconstruction have been shown to be markedly impaired by the presence of concurrent meniscal injury.

The functional importance of the menisci in vivo has been proven unequivocally by clinical studies documenting the long-term results after meniscectomy (Fairbank et al.).

Burke et al. demonstrated that pressure distribution patterns within the knee were less affected by partial meniscectomy leaving the peripheral portion of the meniscus intact, than by total meniscectomy.

Many meniscal tears are irreparable, in which case partial or total meniscectomy is inevitable.

Possible solutions to such cases may lie with techniques such as meniscal allograft transplantation after total meniscectomy or partial meniscal replacement with collagen scaffolds after partial meniscectomy.

The Meniscus: Basic Science

2

H. Pereira, J. Silva-Correia, J. M. Oliveira, R. L. Reis and J. Espregueira-Mendes

2.1 Introduction

The menisci are semilunar discs of fibrocartilaginous tissue which play critical roles in knee joint biomechanics [1]. Despite, it have been described in the past as nearly useless, with perhaps some minor roles on joint nutrition and stabilization [2]. These complex structures are primarily composed of an interlacing network of collagen fibers (predominantly type I collagen) interposed with cells, and an extracellular matrix (ECM) of proteoglycans and glycoproteins.

Menisci are placed within each knee, between the correspondent lateral and medial femoral condyles and tibial plateaux. It has been now recognized that its removal determines deleterious joint consequences, particularly on the long term [3].

Due to the pivotal role of meniscus in maintaining knee homeostasis and proper joint functioning/stability, novel regenerative treatments have been attempted to develop as an alternative to traditional repair procedures or meniscectomy.

The basic science knowledge concerning human meniscus require re-appreciation given the overturn on therapeutic approach, i.e. from meniscectomy to preservation or substitution; and the nearly universal arthroscopic surgical approach opposing to open surgery.

The biological characterization of this tissue, although not yet completely accomplished, has evolved significantly in the last few years. This is true concerning recognition of different cellular populations, understanding its ultrastructure [4], cells and extracellular matrix segmental distributions, biomechanical properties, biologic interactions and mechanism for triggering the response to injury.

H. Pereira · J. Silva-Correia · J. M. Oliveira · R. L. Reis · J. Espregueira-Mendes (✉)
Clínica Espregueira-Mendes, Estádio do Dragão, Porto, 4350-415, Portugal
e-mail: jem@espregueira.com

H. Pereira
e-mail: heldermdpereira@gmail.com

R. Verdonk et al. (eds.), *Meniscal Transplantation*,
DOI: 10.1007/978-3-642-38106-5_2, © ISAKOS 2013

2.2 Anatomy and Biomechanics

In early eighties, a biomechanical study stated the importance of medial meniscus on load transfer. Kurosawa et al. showed that total meniscectomy reduces the total contact area by a third to a half in the fully extended knee [5]. Another report stated its major importance in load transfer and the possible consequences of meniscal excision, not only in articular surface, but also on the subchondral bone, proximal tibia's trabecular bone and cortex [6]. The menisci are not firmly fixed on the tibia and follow knee anteroposterior translation during joint motion. Due to its anatomical features (including stronger attachment to medial collateral ligament), the medial is less mobile. In the stable knee (functioning central pivot ligaments) the medial meniscus has little participation on anterior tibial displacement constraint. The anterior cruciate ligament stops anterior knee motion prior to significant contact of femoral condyle with posterior horn of medial meniscus and tibial plateau [7].

There are major differences between both femorotibial compartments on knee joint to be considered. Lateral tibial plateau is prone to have a more convex shape, opposing to concave shape on medial compartment [1, 7]. This fact helps to understand that the loss of the lateral meniscus leads to major diminishment on femorotibial congruence. Furthermore, according to Walker et al., the lateral meniscus carries most of load transfer on lateral compartment, while in the medial force transmission is distributed between the exposed cartilage surfaces and respective meniscus [8]. *In vitro* trials stated about 70 and 50 % of load transmission through the corresponding menisci in the lateral and medial compartment respectively [9].

Regarding gross morphology, medial meniscus resembles a "C", whereas lateral meniscus is more sharply curved (Fig. 2.1). There is a great variability in medial meniscus anterior horn insertion types, but insertions of the lateral meniscus are less

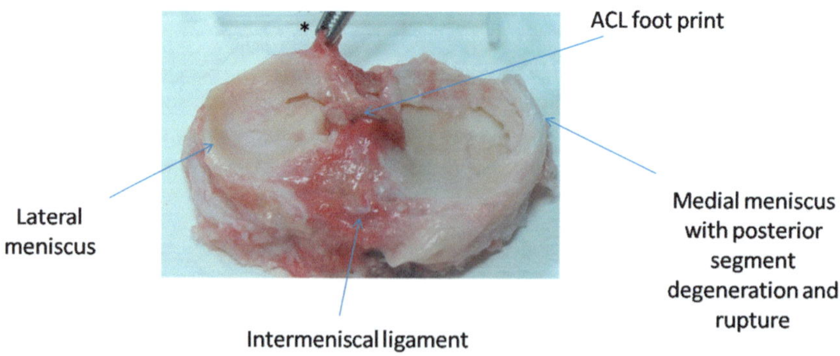

Fig. 2.1 Human specimen photo with menisci in place; ligament of Humphrey also present (attached with forceps*)

variable and quite closer [10–12]. These variants must be taken into account when performing any kind of meniscus substitution.

The biomechanical response of the menisci to loads acting on tibiofemoral joints result from their macro-geometry, their fine architecture and their insertional ligaments. The collagen bundles of the superficial layer are randomly orientated mimicking articular hyaline cartilage [13] (Fig. 2.2). This way it lowers friction between menisci, femur and tibia during joint motion.

In the bulk of the meniscal tissue, under these surface layers, two distinct regions of different collagen fibers are present: the inner one-third bundles have a radial pattern, whereas the outer two-thirds are oriented in a circumferential manner.

Accordingly, it has been suggested that the inner third may function in compression and the outer two-thirds function in tension. Furthermore, some radially-orientated collagen fibers can also be found within the bulk of the meniscal tissue acting as "tie fibers", and resisting longitudinal splitting of the circumferential collagen bundles [14].

Viscoelastic behavior (rubber-like at high loading frequencies; at lower frequencies viscous dissipation occurs) of the meniscus relates with ECM composition (not much dependent of collagen content; higher with increasing glucosaminoglycans (GAGs) content and lower with increasing water content. Accordingly, regional variations can be observed in terms of viscoelastic properties [15]. It has been demonstrated a regional and zonal variation in glycosaminoglycan coverage, size, and cellular density in animal meniscal tissue [16]. Similar studies on human tissue have been required, particularly in the era of Tissue Engineering aiming to replicate menisci in laboratory for clinical application [17]. Pereira et al. have recently presented the first biomechanical segmental characterization of fresh human meniscus [18].

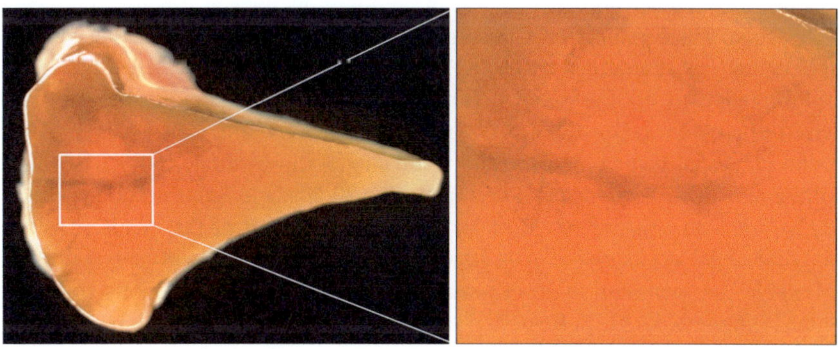

Fig. 2.2 Stereomicroscopy images of human meniscus where it is possible to observe the bundles

The anterior intermeniscal ligament (or transverse geniculate) connects the anterior fibers of the anterior horns of medial and lateral menisci. Its prevalence is estimated around 60 % and its functional relevance remains unclear [19].

Two ligaments are known to connect the posterior horn of the lateral meniscus to the lateral side of the medial condyle of the femur-meniscofemoral ligaments.

The ligament of Humphrey runs anterior to the posterior cruciate ligament (PCL), while the ligament of Wrisberg runs posterior to the PCL. Their estimated prevalence is 74 % for Humphrey ligament, 69 % for Wrisberg ligament, and both ligaments found together in around 50 % of knees [20].

The functional relevance of these ligaments has been demonstrated by Gupte et al., who demonstrated that menisco-femoral ligaments contributed 28 % to the total force resisting posterior drawer at 90° of flexion in the intact knee, and 70.1 % in the PCL-deficient knee [21]. Probably this issue will remain a research topic aiming to improve meniscal repair or replacement techniques.

2.3 Extracellular Matrix and Cellularity

Considering composition by wet weight, the meniscus has high water content (72 %). The remaining 28 % consists of an organic component, mostly ECM and cells [22]. Collagens comprise the majority (75 %) of the organic matter, followed by GAGs (17 %), DNA (2 %), adhesion glycoproteins (<1 %), and elastin (<1 %) [22, 23]. These proportions vary according to age, injury, or pathological conditions [24].

Collagen is the main fibrillar component of the meniscus. Different collagen types exist in various quantities in each region of meniscus. In the red–red zone, type I collagen is predominant (80 % composition in dry weight), but other collagen variants (e.g., type II, III, IV, VI, and XVIII) are present at less than 1 %. In the white–white zone, collagen makes up to 70 % dry weight, of which 60 % is type II collagen and 40 % is type I collagen [25].

Elastin is another fibrillar component, although its relevance is not completely understood. The combination of mature and immature elastin fibers has been found in very low concentrations (<0.6 %) in the adult meniscus [26, 27].

Proteoglycans are the major component of ECM. These molecules are comprised of a core protein which is decorated with GAGs. The main types of GAGs found in normal human meniscal tissue are chondoitin-6-sulfate (60 %), dermatan sulfate (20–30 %), chondroitin-4-sulfate (10–20 %), and keratin sulfate (15 %) [23]. Aggrecan constitutes the major large proteoglycan of the meniscus, while biglycan and decorin are the main small proteoglycans [28]. Their main function is to enable the meniscus to absorb water, whose confinement supports the tissue under compression [22]. Regional variation of these molecules has also been observed, with the inner two-thirds containing a relatively higher proportion of proteoglycans than the outer one-third [28].

Adhesion glycoproteins are also important components of the meniscus matrix, as they serve as a link between ECM components and cells. The main adhesion glycoproteins present in the human meniscus are fibronectin, thrombospondin, and type VI collagen [29].

Considering shape classification and territorial ECM, chondrocyte-like, fibroblast-like, and intermediate cells were identified in the meniscus [30]. Classification of meniscus cells is controversial and different terms are being used (i.e. fibrocytes, fibroblasts, meniscus cells, fibrochondrocytes, and chondrocytes) [31].

It is apparent that outer zone cells have an oval, fusiform shape and are similar in appearance and behavior to fibroblasts. Thus, they may be described as fibroblast-like cells [4]. These cells also display long cell extensions, which facilitate communication with other cells and the ECM. The matrix surrounding the cells is mainly comprised of type I collagen, with small percentages of glycoproteins and types III and V collagen [32].

In contrast, cells in the inner portion have rounded appearance and are embedded in an ECM comprising largely type II collagen intermingled with a smaller but significant amount of type I collagen and a higher concentration of GAGs. This relative abundance of type II collagen and aggrecan in the inner region is more reminiscent of hyaline articular cartilage. Therefore, cells in this region are classified as fibrochondrocytes or chondrocyte-like cells [4].

A third cell population has also been recognized in the superficial zone of the meniscus. These cells have somewhat peculiar morphology, i.e. are flattened, fusiform and lack the cell extensions. It has been suggested that these might be specific progenitor cells with more regenerative capacities [33].

Outer meniscus cells seem to migrate quicker and exhibited lower adhesion strengths as compared to inner meniscus cells [34].

Meniscus cells isolated from outer (vascular), inner (avascular), and horn (mixed) can be induced towards chondrogenic, adipogenic and osteogenic lineages. Outer cells are more plastic and can also go to osteogenesis [35]. The distribution of different cells in the meniscus architecture (segments and zones) has recently been focus of research and it is a relevant insight in the ambitious goal of achieving a tissue engineered implant [18].

2.4 Vascularization and Innervation

Three classical zones according to vascularization continue to be used as references: red–red; red–white e white–white (Fig. 2.3a, b) perfectly shows the blood vessels at red–red zone, which arise mainly from medial and lateral inferior and middle geniculate arteries. Radial branches from a perimeniscal plexus enter the

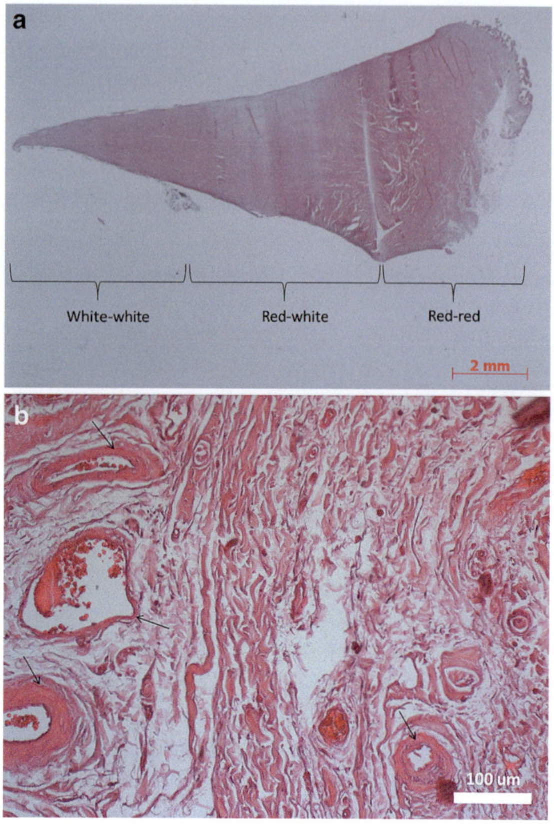

Fig. 2.3 Microscopy image of a section of human meniscus stained with haematoxylin and eosin (**a**), and respective magnification of red–red zone where it is possible to observe the blood vessels (*black arrows*) (**b**)

meniscus at intervals, with a richer supply to the anterior and posterior horns [36]. Vessels supplying the body are limited to the meniscus periphery with a variable penetration of 10–30 % for medial meniscus and 10–25 % for lateral one, except in the fetus. There is an avascular area adjacent to the popliteus tendon [37].

The perimeniscal tissue is richly innervated. Most nerves are associated with vessels. Smaller nerves and axons run radially in convoluted patterns. Single axons course through the perimeniscal tissue, and many nerves are seen in the interstitial tissue of the peripheral zone of the meniscus and in the anterior and posterior horns. The inner menisci core has no nerve fibers [36].

Studies of the vascular and nerve supply of the meniscus in humans have potentially important clinical applications. It has been established that meniscal vasculature is related to the ability of meniscal tissue to heal well, although some healing of meniscal tissue has also been described in avascular portions of the meniscus.

In the fetus, the vascular supply is more extensive, with vessels extending to the inner one-third. There is also a significant nerve supply that is similar in distribution to the vascular supply.

2.5 Conclusions

Progressive insights in meniscus structure, biology and biomechanical properties are uprising. Such knowledge plays a determinant role in the development of further therapeutic options for full repair of these structures known to be critical to the long lasting physiological functioning of the knee joint.

References

1. McDermott ID, Masouros SD, Amis AA (2008) Biomechanics of the menisci of the knee. Curr Orthopaed 22:193–201
2. Smillie IS (1972) Injuries of the knee joint, 4th edn. Churcill Livingstone, Edinburgh
3. Fayard JM, Pereira H, Servien E, Lustig S, Neyret P (2010) Meniscectomy global results-complications. Springer-Verlag, Berlin Heidelberg
4. Verdonk PC, Forsyth RG, Wang J et al (2005) Characterisation of human knee meniscus cell phenotype. Osteoarthritis Cartilage 13:548–560
5. Kurosawa H, Fukubayashi T, Nakajima H (1980) Load-bearing mode of the knee joint: physical behavior of the knee joint with or without menisci. Clin Orthop Relat Res 283–290
6. Fukubayashi T, Kurosawa H (1980) The contact area and pressure distribution pattern of the knee. A study of normal and osteoarthrotic knee joints. Acta Orthop Scand 51:871–879
7. Levy IM, Torzilli PA, Warren RF (1982) The effect of medial meniscectomy on anterior-posterior motion of the knee. J Bone Joint Surg Am 64:883–888
8. Walker PS, Hajek JV (1972) The load-bearing area in the knee joint. J Biomech 5:581–589
9. Bourne RB, Finlay JB, Papadopoulos P, Andreae P (1984) The effect of medial meniscectomy on strain distribution in the proximal part of the tibia. J Bone Joint Surg Am 66:1431–1437
10. Brody JM, Hulstyn MJ, Fleming BC, Tung GA (2007) The meniscal roots: gross anatomic correlation with 3-T MRI findings. AJR Am J Roentgenol 188:W446–W450
11. Wilmes P, Pape D, Kohn D, Seil R (2007) The reproducibility of radiographic measurement of lateral meniscus horn position. Arthroscopy 23:1079–1086
12. Wilmes P, Anagnostakos K, Weth C, Kohn D, Seil R (2008) The reproducibility of radiographic measurement of medial meniscus horn position. Arthroscopy 24:660–668
13. Beaupre A, Choukroun R, Guidouin R, Garneau R, Gerardin H, Cardou A (1986) Knee menisci. Correlation between microstructure and biomechanics. Clin Orthop Relat Res 72–75
14. Bullough PG, Munuera L, Murphy J, Weinstein AM (1970) The strength of the menisci of the knee as it relates to their fine structure. J Bone Joint Surg Br 52:564–567
15. Bursac P, Arnoczky S, York A (2009) Dynamic compressive behavior of human meniscus correlates with its extra-cellular matrix composition. Biorheology 46:227–237
16. Killian ML, Lepinski NM, Haut RC, Haut Donahue TL (2010) Regional and zonal histo-morphological characteristics of the lapine menisci. Anat Rec (Hoboken) 293:1991–2000
17. Pereira H, Frias AM, Oliveira JM, Espregueira-Mendes J, Reis RL (2011) Tissue engineering and regenerative medicine strategies in meniscus lesions. Arthroscopy 27:1706–1719
18. Pereira H, Frias AM, Caridade SG et al (2011) Cellular and biomechanical segmental characterization of human meniscus. Osteoarthritis Cartilage 19:S205

19. Kohn D, Moreno B (1995) Meniscus insertion anatomy as a basis for meniscus replacement: a morphological cadaveric study. Arthroscopy 11:96–103
20. Gupte CM, Smith A, McDermott ID, Bull AM, Thomas RD, Amis AA (2002) Meniscofemoral ligaments revisited. Anatomical study, age correlation and clinical implications. J Bone Joint Surg Br 84:846–851
21. Gupte CM, Bull AM, Thomas RD, Amis AA (2003) The meniscofemoral ligaments: secondary restraints to the posterior drawer. Analysis of anteroposterior and rotary laxity in the intact and posterior-cruciate-deficient knee. J Bone Joint Surg Br 85:765–773
22. Makris EA, Hadidi P, Athanasiou KA (2011) The knee meniscus: structure-function, pathophysiology, current repair techniques, and prospects for regeneration. Biomaterials 32:7411–7431
23. Herwig J, Egner E, Buddecke E (1984) Chemical changes of human knee joint menisci in various stages of degeneration. Ann Rheum Dis 43:635–640
24. Sweigart MA, Athanasiou KA (2001) Toward tissue engineering of the knee meniscus. Tissue Eng 7:111–129
25. Cheung HS (1987) Distribution of type I, II, III and V in the pepsin solubilized collagens in bovine menisci. Connect Tissue Res 16:343–356
26. McDevitt CA, Webber RJ (1992) The ultrastructure and biochemistry of meniscal cartilage. Clin Orthop Relat Res 252:8–18
27. Ghosh P, Taylor TK (1987) The knee joint meniscus. A fibrocartilage of some distinction. Clin Orthop Relat Res 52–63
28. Scott PG, Nakano T, Dodd CM (1997) Isolation and characterization of small proteoglycans from different zones of the porcine knee meniscus. Biochim Biophys Acta 1336:254–262
29. Miller RR, McDevitt CA (1991) Thrombospondin in ligament, meniscus and intervertebral disc. Biochim Biophys Acta 1115:85–88
30. Ghadially FN, Thomas I, Yong N, Lalonde JM (1978) Ultrastructure of rabbit semilunar cartilages. J Anat 125:499–517
31. Nakata K, Shino K, Hamada M et al (2001) Human meniscus cell: characterization of the primary culture and use for tissue engineering. Clin Orthop Relat Res S208–S218
32. Melrose J, Smith S, Cake M, Read R, Whitelock J (2005) Comparative spatial and temporal localisation of perlecan, aggrecan and type I, II and IV collagen in the ovine meniscus: an ageing study. Histochem Cell Biol 124:225–235
33. Van der Bracht H, Verdonk R, Verbruggen G, Elewaut D, Verdonk P (2007) Cell based meniscus tissue engineering. In: Ashammakhi N, Reis RL, Chiellini E (eds) Topics in Tissue Engineering
34. Gunja NJ, Dujari D, Chen A, Luengo A, Fong JV, Hung CT (2012) Migration responses of outer and inner meniscus cells to applied direct current electric fields. J Orthop Res 30:103–111
35. Mauck RL, Martinez-Diaz GJ, Yuan X, Tuan RS (2007) Regional multilineage differentiation potential of meniscal fibrochondrocytes: implications for meniscus repair. Anat Rec (Hoboken) 290:48–58
36. Brian D, Mackenzie WG, Shim SS, Leung G (1985) The vascular and nerve supply of the human meniscus. Arthroscopy 1:58–62
37. Arnoczky SP, Warren RF (1982) Microvasculature of the human meniscus. Am J Sports Med 10:90–95

Organisation: Type of Grafts—Conservation—Regulation

3

Ch. Delloye, T. Schubert and O. Cornu

3.1 Introduction

Joint degeneration following complete meniscus removal has been documented and recognized as a major cause of osteoarthritis [1–5]. The meniscus at the knee has been shown to serve various functions such as load distribution, shock absorption, joint stability, knee proprioception and joint lubrication. A deficient meniscus implies a decrease of surface contact area with a subsequent increase of contact pressure, leading to wear and gradual disappearance of cartilage within a decade [6–9]. The basic principle underlying meniscal transplantation is to restore the joint anatomy and to relocate an implant that will serve and perform in a similar fashion as the original one.

An allograft should delay or better still, prevent osteoarthritis of the knee.

The demand for meniscal allografts has recently increased because of the improvements in graft fixation and the extended indications for meniscus allografting.

Limitations to musculoskeletal tissue donation and donor age contribute to the shortage of available meniscal tissue. Optimal handling and fixation of a meniscus allograft during surgery will avoid tissue wasting and improve the surgical outcome.

Ch. Delloye · T. Schubert · O. Cornu (✉)
Cliniques Universitaires St Luc, Louvain La Neuve, Department of Orthop and Trauma, Brussels, Belgium
e-mail: Olivier.cornu@orto.ucl.ac.be

Ch. Delloye
e-mail: delloye@orto.ucl.ac.be

T. Schubert
e-mail: T.shubert@ orto.ucl.ac.be

R. Verdonk et al. (eds.), *Meniscal Transplantation*,
DOI: 10.1007/978-3-642-38106-5_3, © ISAKOS 2013

3.1.1 Tissue Banking Organization

Meniscus transplantation deals with human tissues and, as such, is regulated by the European directive on human tissue, which sets the standards of quality and safety for the donation, procurement, testing, processing, preservation, storage and distribution of human tissues and cells [10–12]. Most large tissue banks are involved throughout the whole process from harvest to graft delivery [13, 14].

3.1.2 Donor Selection

3.1.2.1 Consent

The procurement of any human tissue is framed by European directives on human tissue, covering donation, donor selection and tissue safety. In each country, the European directive must be translated into a national law of at least the same level of requirements. Each country has the possibility to reinforce one or more legal aspects. A national authority controls tissue banking activities in each European country.

Menisci are procured from young adult organ donors. Consent for tissue retrieval is obtained according to the national law and European regulations.

In Belgium, the consent is based on donor presumed consent. Tissue harvesting is allowed only if the potential donor is not registered with a national registry. Nevertheless, informed consent from the next of kin will always be sought,

Anonymity between donor and recipient is a key principle, whereas traceability is maintained by a unique donor coding number [12].

3.1.2.2 Donor Selection

Donor suitability is determined in compliance with the standards and guidelines developed by European or national authorities, or tissue banking associations such as the American Association of Tissue Banks (AATB) and the European Association of MusculoSkeletal Transplantation (EAMST). Those standards list a series of conditions that might indicate a donor at risk for disease transmission [11, 12, 15–17]. Thorough examination of the medical files and donor physical assessment are imperative.

European standards differ from American ones in two specific points [10, 11, 15, 16]. A past history of cancer is an exclusion criterion in Europe but not necessarily in the United States. In Europe, the donor's body must be refrigerated within six hours for a procurement to occur within 24 h after death, whereas in the United States an interval not exceeding 15 h prior to body cooling can be accepted before procurement.The donor is screened for disease transmission prior to tissue harvesting. If the potential donor has been transfused with a large volume (>2,000 ml) of blood, blood components or plasma volume expanders within 48 h prior to death, a pretransfusion blood sample is required for testing, because dilution of donor plasma carries a risk of false—negative results.

HIV-1 and 2 (two antibodies tests and *P24* antigen detection), HTLV-1 (antibodies), hepatitis B (surface antigen *HBs* and core antibody *HBc*), hepatitis C (antibodies) and syphilis (antibodies) are systematically screened. Additional safety measures can be taken to screen for potentially false-negative results during the incubation period of a virus, by using nucleic acid testing for hepatitis viruses and HIV (NAT). This type of assay allows significant reduction of the serological window period [17–19]. Furthermore, another safety feedback is possible for tissues procured from an organ donor as organ recipients can be screened for disease transmission three months after having been grafted [17].

Blood cultures are recommended because they reflect the bacterial quality of the harvested tissue [20, 21].

During and after harvesting, samples of the procured tissues are placed in a thioglycolate broth culture medium in order to exclude bacteriological contamination [14, 22]. They are cultured for aerobic and anaerobic bacteriae and fungi for at least seven days.

3.1.2.3 Harvesting

Harvesting from a multiorgan donor is performed under sterile conditions in the operating theatre by a team of three to four trained individuals, one being an orthopaedic surgeon. When selecting viable meniscal or osteochondral allografts, the donor should preferably be under 45 years of age. Close examination at the time of procurement will determine the quality of the surface of the cartilage and of the meniscus. In daily practice, donor age is certainly not the main critical factor: posttraumatic or osteoarthritic changes may be present in younger patients, whereas suitable cartilage or meniscus might sometimes be found in donors above the age limit of 45 years.

At our institution, a 1 cm-thick section of the tibial plateau is removed (Fig. 3.1). Then, the plateau is in its central aspect separated into two parts, taking care not to damage the insertions of the menisci (Fig. 3.2).

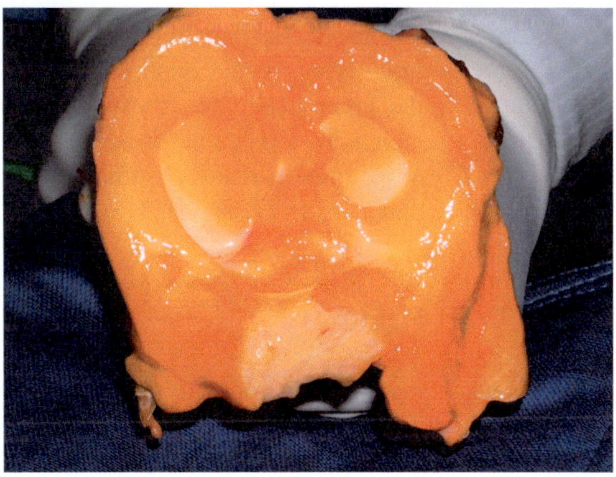

Fig. 3.1 Menisci harvested. Aspect prior to bone sawing

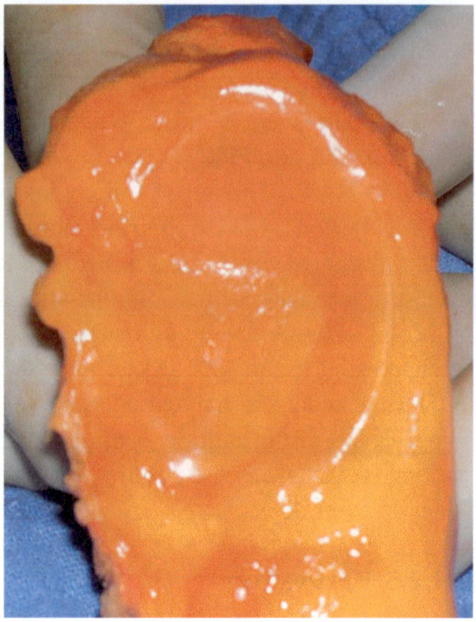

Fig. 3.2 Meniscus harvested with its osseous support

3.1.2.4 Risks and Recommendations

Bone and tissue allografts are capable of transmitting virus and contaminating the recipient [23–28]. The risk of viral disease transmission through tissue is very low, provided that the guidelines for donor selection have been strictly followed and that the donor has been screened by medical history-taking and blood testing. For HIV the theoretical risk of transmission has been evaluated to be less than one in a million, and for HCV one in 200,000 for an unprocessed tissue from a selected and serologically screened donor [29–31].

For a processed tissue such as cancellous bone that has been subjected to thorough saline washing and solvent-detergent exposure with a final irradiation, the theoretical risk is much lower, with an average decrease of two orders of magnitude [26, 30].

The surgeon using the graft must verify the bacteriological and serological results himself and inform the patient of the use of an allograft.

ABO blood group typing is not required prior to a bone or soft-tissue grafting procedure. On the other hand, the Rhesus factor has to be determined if the recipient is a female with a potential of becoming pregnant [32, 33]. It has been shown that 0.5 ml of bone marrow is sufficient to induce Rhesus immunity in a Rhesus-negative patient. Soft tissue such as meniscus does not carry this risk.

3.1.3 Graft Sizing

Sizing is usually based on peroperative measurements and standard X-rays.

For peroperative sizing of the graft, the anteroposterior and lateromedial dimensions are measured, as well as the width of the meniscus at its anterior,

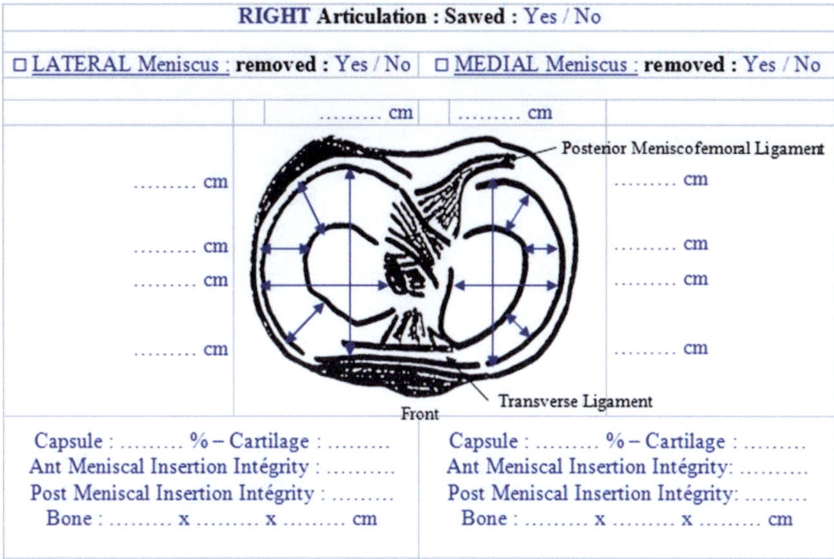

Fig. 3.3 Graft sizing. Standard sizing chart used in the operating theatre

medial and posterior parts [34]. All measures are recorded on standardized charts and are catalogued in our tissue bank inventory, providing a wide range of meniscal transplants (Fig. 3.3).

Standard X-rays are difficult to obtain. If true anteroposterior or lateral images are lacking, the inaccuracy of the measurements is significantly increased (Figs. 3.4 and 3.5) [35].

Magnetic resonance imaging (MRI) is not used by bone banks because its superiority has not been clearly demonstrated. Moreover, MRI is not easily applicable in a routine tissue bank protocol or pretransplantation planning [35–37].

A successful transplantation requires precise matching of the size of the donor meniscus and the recipient. The use of digital imaging during procurement might be helpful [38, 39].

3.1.4 Types of Grafts

According to the preservation method, four types of allografts are distinguished : fresh menisci, frozen menisci with or without cryoprotectants, and freeze-dried menisci. While fresh and cryopreserved grafts may still contain some viable cells at the time of transplantation, freeze-dried and deep-frozen ones are nonviable and are as such considered to be acellular material [40, 41].

Fresh meniscus is used for viable meniscus allografting. For maximal viability of the meniscus to be preserved, procurement should be within 12 h after death.

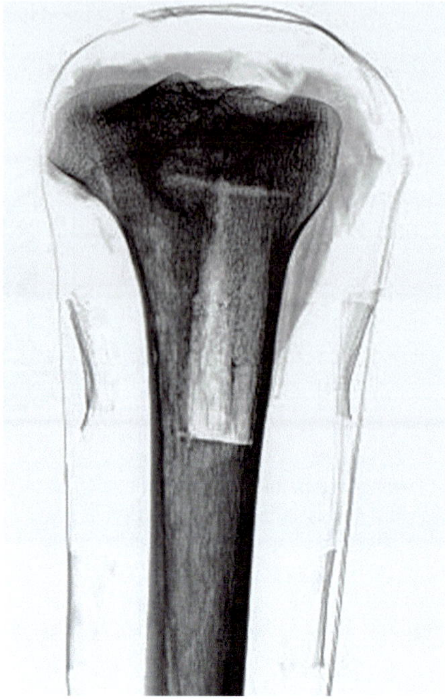

Fig. 3.4 Standard AP view of a procured tibia with menisci

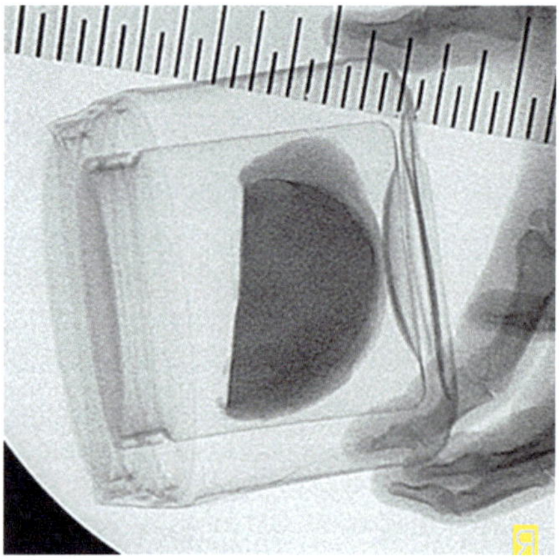

Fig. 3.5 Frontal view of a harvested meniscus

After harvesting, the grafts are transported in a sterile saline solution and placed in a culture medium containing 20 % of recipient serum. The graft material is stored at 37 °C in a constant controlled environment [41, 42]. Postimplantation viability of fresh grafts has been documented [41, 43]. Because cultured meniscus does produce the components of the extracellular matrix in vitro, it can be expected to perform similarly in vivo. However, the duration of this cellular function in vivo remains unknown. In a goat model, DNA probing showed that cells from fresh and viable meniscus did not survive for more than one month [44]. However, Verdonk et al. were able to demonstrate some donor cell survival 64 months after transplantation [43].

Recipients of a fresh meniscal allograft do not require immunosuppression, but the importance of the recipient's immune response to the clinical outcome remains unknown [45]. So far, no clear benefit has been shown of a viable meniscal allograft compared to a frozen-preserved one.

Cryopreserved meniscal allografts are tissues that are immerged in a solution containing a cryoprotective agent such as dimethyl sulfoxide (DMSO), a culture medium and an antiseptic agent. After impregnation, the graft is gradually frozen in a controlled fashion to minimize cellular lesions during freezing. Storage temperature is at −196 °C. Even if this type of cryopreserved graft may still contain viable cells after thawing, their long- term survival remains questionable [46].

Freshly frozen allografts are soaked in a saline solution containing an antibiotic (rifampicin, 1.2 g/l) after harvesting. Subsequently, they are packaged in a sterile fashion and stored in a mechanical freezer at −80 °C. These grafts can be preserved for as long as five years. At surgery, they are again soaked in an antibiotic solution, e.g. rifampicin, which will be gradually released from the implant for at least three weeks after the operation in a similar fashion as demonstrated for bone [30, 47].

Freezing a tissue without other physical treatment such as irradiation does not alter the original mechanical properties, whatever the freezing temperature [48, 49].

The maximal storage period of human deep-frozen tissue is limited to five years in Europe [17].

Freeze-dried allografts: lyophilization or freeze-drying, which consists of drying a tissue under vacuum and freezing conditions, is a suitable method to preserve cellular viability if cryoprotective solutions are used, as for vaccine production. Lyophilization without cryoprotection leaves nonviable dried tissue [30, 50]. Freeze-drying is just a preservation method and as such, not a sterilant.

Freeze-drying is beneficial from a logistical standpoint, because the dried tissue can be stored at ambient room temperature. In addition, from an immunological standpoint, lyophilization has been demonstrated to be superior to freezing, because freeze-dried tissue does not elicit an immune response, at least not in experimental conditions [51].

Because sterile freeze-drying of tissues is difficult, further irradiation at 25 Kgy is usually associated. In a clinical setting, the dried tissue is also irradiated for final sterilization. This combined process of lyophilization and irradiation appears to be detrimental to the tissue, because it results in a profound alteration of the mechanical properties and the extracellular matrix. From a clinical standpoint, freeze-dried and irradiated meniscal allografts are not suitable for transplantation [52–54].

Table 3.1 Allograft use algorithm

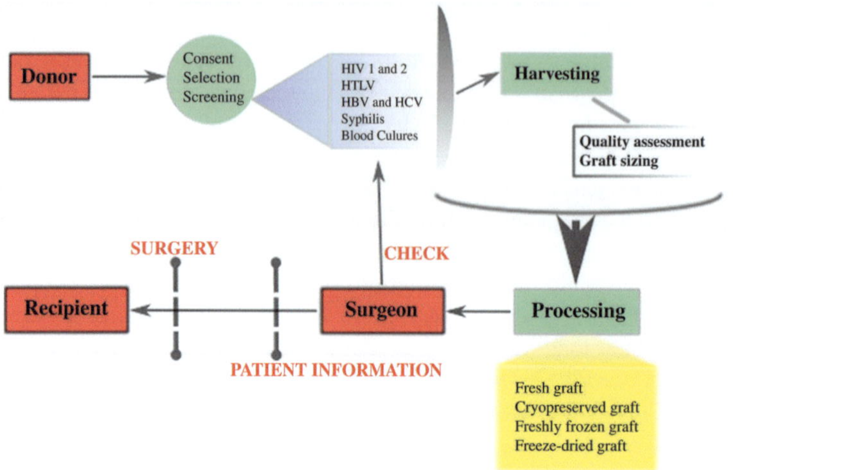

3.1.5 Data from Our Bank

Our bank has always worked with freshly frozen tissues. Table 3.1 summarizes the path followed by any tissue from donor to recipient. Over the last years, the demand for meniscal allografts has substantially increased, since the year 2000 even 20-fold, with an annual delivery rate of 45 menisci in 2006 and 2007. We advocate the deep-freezing method for several reasons: (1) it does not affect the mechanical properties of the tissue; (2) even if the material is nonviable at surgery, experimental conditions have shown a rapid recolonization of the implant by host cells; (3) it allows storage for five years; (4) it requires minimal tissue handling compared to cultured tissue; and (5) it allows the surgeon to schedule the time of surgery himself. In 2007, we reviewed 69 fresh-frozen meniscal allografts procured by our tissue bank, with a follow-up of two years. Of these 69 grafts, 60 % had been secured by peripheral suturing, 22 % with one bone plug and 18 % with two bone plugs. Using psychometric scores for knee evaluation, an increase of four points on the Tegner activity scale [55] was achieved, corresponding with a 65 % improvement after allograft surgery. The mean Lysholm score [55] increased from 72 preoperatively to 90 at the last postoperative visit. As for patient satisfaction, we noted 90 % of excellent results and 8 % of intermediate results, while 2 % of patients were disappointed by the surgery. We encountered four complications: three tears and one infection.

Apparently, freshly frozen allografts can be safely and reliably used for meniscal transplantation.

References

1. Allen PR, Denham RA, Swan AV (1984) Late degenerative changes after meniscectomy. Factors affecting the knee after operation. J Bone Joint Surg Br 66:666–671
2. Fairbank TJ (1948) Knee joint changes after meniscectomy. J Bone Joint Surg Br 30-B: 664–670
3. Johnson RJ, Kettelkamp DB, Clark W et al (1974) Factors effecting late results after meniscectomy. J Bone Joint Surg Am 56:719–729
4. McNicholas MJ, Rowley DI, McGurty D et al (2000) Total meniscectomy in adolescence: a thirty-year follow-up. J Bone Joint Surg Br 82-B:217–221
5. Tapper EM, Hoover NW (1969) Late results after meniscectomy. J Bone Joint Surg Am 51:517–526
6. Bourne RB, Finlay JB, Papadopoulos P et al (1984) The effect of medial meniscectomy on strain distribution in the proximal part of the tibia. J Bone Joint Surg Am 66:1431–1437
7. Krause WR, Pope MH, Johnson RJ et al (1976) Mechanical changes in the knee after meniscectomy. J Bone Joint Surg Am 58:599–604
8. Levy IM, Torzilli PA, Warren RF (1982) The effect of medial meniscectomy on anterior-posterior motion of the knee. J Bone Joint Surg Am 64:883–888
9. Shoemaker SC, Markolf KL (1986) The role of the meniscus in the anterior-posterior stability of the loaded anterior cruciate-deficient knee. Effects of partial versus total excision. J Bone Joint Surg Am 68:71–79
10. Official journal of European Union (2004) Directive 2004/23/EC of the European Parliament and of the council of 31 march 2004 on setting standards of quality and safety for the donation, procurement, testing, processing, preservation, storage and distribution of human tissues and cells
11. Official Journal of European Union (2006) Commission Directive 2006/17/EC of 8 February 2006 as regards certain technical requirements for the donation, procurement and testing of human tissues and cells
12. Official journal of European Union (2006) Commission Directive 2006/86/EC of 24 October 2006 as regards traceability requirements, notification of serious adverse reactions and events and certain technical requirements for the coding, processing, preservation, storage and distribution of human tissues and cells
13. Friedlaender GE, Mankin HJ (1981) Bone banking: current methods and suggested guidelines. Instr Course Lect 30:36–55
14. Tomford WW, Doppelt SH, Mankin HJ et al (1983) 1983 bone bank procedures. Clin Orthop Relat Res 174:15–21
15. American Association of Tissue Banks (1984) Standards for tissue banking, 1st edn. American Association of Tissue Banks, Arlington
16. American Association of Tissue Banks (2008) Standards for tissue banking, 12th edn. American Association of Tissue Banks, McLean
17. European association of musculoskeletal transplantation (EAMST) and European association of tissue banks (EATB) (1997) Common standards for musculoskeletal tissue banking. Vienna, Austria
18. Burtonboy G, Delloye C (1996) Polymerase chain reaction in cadaveric blood and tissues. Transplant Proc 28:2927–2928
19. Lelie PN, Zaaijer HL, Cuypers HT (1996) Risk of virus transmission by tissue, blood, and plasma products. Transplant Proc 28:2939–2939
20. Deijkers RL, Bloem RM, Petit PL et al (1997) Contamination of bone allografts: analysis of incidence and predisposing factors. J Bone Joint Surg Br 79:161–166
21. Deijkers RL, Vehmeyer SB, Veen MR et al (1995) 5-year experience with a central bone bank. Ned Tijdschr Geneeskd 139:622–626

22. Tomford WW, Thongphasuk J, Mankin HJ et al (1990) Frozen musculoskeletal allografts. A study of the clinical incidence and causes of infection associated with their use. J Bone Joint Surg Am 72:1137–1143
23. Buck BE, Resnick L, Shah et al (1990) Human immunodeficiency virus cultured from bone. Implications for transplantation. Clin Orthop Relat Res 251: 249–253
24. Campbell DG, Li P, Oakeshott RD (1996) Hiv infection of human cartilage. J Bone Joint Surg Br 78:22–25
25. Center for Disease Control (1988) Transmission of hiv through bone transplantation: case report and public health recommendations. MMWR Morb Mortal Wkly Rep 37:597–599
26. Conrad EU, Gretch DR, Obermeyer KR et al (1995) Transmission of the hepatitis-c virus by tissue transplantation. J Bone Joint Surg Am 77:214–224
27. Simonds RJ, Holmberg SD, Hurwitz RL et al (1992) Transmission of human immunodeficiency virus type 1 from a seronegative organ and tissue donor. N Engl J Med 326:726–732
28. Tomford WW (1995) Transmission of disease through transplantation of musculoskeletal allografts. J Bone Joint Surg Am 77:1742–1754
29. Buck BE, Malinin TI, Brown MD (1989) Bone transplantation and human immunodeficiency virus. An estimate of risk of acquired immunodeficiency syndrome. Clin Orthop Relat Res 240:129–136
30. Delloye C, Naets B, Cnockaert N et al (2004) Harvest, storage and microbiological safety of bone allografts. In: Marcel Dekker Inc. Impaction bone grafting in revision arthroplasty. New-York
31. Eggen BM, Nordb SA (1992) Transmission of HCV by organ transplantation. N Engl J Med 326:411
32. Jensen TT (1987) Rhesus immunization after bone allografting. A case report. Acta Orthop Scand 58:584–584
33. Johnson CA, Brown BA, Lasky LC (1985) Rh immunization caused by osseous allograft. N Engl J Med 312:121–122
34. McDermott ID, Sharifi F, Bull AMJ et al (2004) An anatomical study of meniscal allograft sizing. Knee Surg Sports Traumatol Arthrosc 12:130–135
35. Shaffer B, Kennedy S, Klimkiewicz J et al (2000) Preoperative sizing of meniscal allografts in meniscus transplantation. Am J Sports Med 28:524–533
36. Haut TL, Hull ML, Howell SM (2000) Use of roentgenography and magnetic resonance imaging to predict meniscal geometry determined with a three-dimensional coordinate digitizing system. J Orthop Res 18:228–237
37. Stone KR, Stoller DW, Irving SG et al (1994) 3D MRI volume sizing of knee meniscus cartilage. Arthroscopy 10:641–644
38. Dienst M, Greis PE, Ellis BJ et al (2007) Effect of lateral meniscal allograft sizing on contact mechanics of the lateral tibial plateau: an experimental study in human cadaveric knee joints. Am J Sports Med 35:34–42
39. Haut TL, Hull ML, Rashid MM et al (2004) The sensitivity of tibiofemoral contact pressure to the size and shape of the lateral and medial menisci. J Orthop Res 22:807–814
40. Cole BJ, Carter TR, Rodeo SA (2003) Allograft meniscal transplantation: background, techniques, and results. Instr Course Lect 52:383–396
41. Verdonk R (2002) Meniscal transplantation. Acta Orthop Belg 68:118–127
42. Verdonk R, Kohn D (1999) Harvest and conservation of meniscal allografts. Scand J Med Sci Sports 9:158–159
43. Verdonk P, Demurie A, Almqvist K et al (2005) Transplantation of viable meniscal allograft. J Bone Joint Surg Am 87:715–724
44. Jackson DW, Whelan J, Simon TM (1993) Cell survival after transplantation of fresh meniscal allografts. DNA probe analysis in a goat model. Am J Sports Med 21:540–550
45. Goble EM, Kohn D, Verdonk R et al (1999) Meniscal substitutes. Human experience. Scand J Med Sci Sports 9:146–157

46. Fabbriciani C, Lucania L, Milano G et al (1997) Meniscal allografts: cryopreservation vs deep-frozen technique. An experimental study in goats. Knee Surg Sports Traumatol Arthrosc 5:124–134
47. Hernigou P, Glorion C, Girard-Pipau F et al (1992) Libération in vitro et in vivo des antibiotiques à partir des greffes osseuse. Rev Chir Orthop 78(suppl 1):217
48. Jackson DW, Grood ES, Wilcox P et al (1988) The effects of processing techniques on the mechanical properties of bone-anterior cruciate ligament-bone allografts. An experimental study in goats. Am J Sports Med 16:101–105
49. Pelker RR, Friedlaender GE, Markham TC et al (1984) Effects of freezing and freeze-drying on the biomechanical properties of rat bone. J Orthop Res 1:405–411
50. Delloye C, De Halleux J, Cornu O et al (1991) Organizational and investigational aspects of bone banking in belgium. Acta Orthop Belg 57(Suppl 2):27–34
51. Friedlaender GE, Strong DM, Sell KW (1976) Studies on the antigenicity of bone. Freeze-dried and deep-frozen bone allografts in rabbits. J Bone Joint Surg Am 58:854–858
52. Milachowski KA, Weismeier K, Wirth CJ (1989) Homologous meniscus transplantation. Experimental and clinical results. Int Orthop 13:1–11
53. Yahia LH, Drouin G, Zukor D (1993) The irradiation effect on the initial mechanical properties of meniscal grafts. Biomed Mater Eng 3:211–221
54. Yahia L, Zukor D (1994) Irradiated meniscal allotransplants of rabbits: study of the mechanical properties at six months postoperation. Acta Orthop Belg 60:210–215
55. Briggs K, Kocher M, Rodkey W et al (2006) Reliability, validity, and responsiveness of the Lysholm knee score and Tegner activity scale for patients with meniscal injury of the knee. J Bone Joint Surg Am 88:698–705
56. Pereira BJ, Milford EL, Kirkman RL et al (1991) Transmission of hepatitis C virus by organ transplantation. N Engl J Med 325:454–460
57. Simonds RJ (1993) Hiv transmission by organ and tissue transplantation. AIDS 7(2):S35–8-S35–8

Surgical Techniques

4

Rene Verdonk

4.1 Open Technique

P. Verdonk[1]
R. Verdonk[2]

4.1.1 Preoperative Considerations

In contrast to the use of deep-frozen allografts, a strict time schedule from harvest to transplantation is mandatory for viable allografts. The transplantation of viable meniscal allografts implies the availability of *viable* donor tissues, cultured in vitro immediately following harvest. Sizing of the graft is critical for correct implantation. For deep-frozen allografts the mediolateral and anteroposterior length of the tibial plateau of the receptor are measured on a calibrated X-ray and transferred to the tissue bank. Since viable meniscal allografting is more limited in size-options due to the fact that there is only 1 donor and a limited number of acceptors, the most appropriate acceptor is chosen based on corresponding donor–acceptor height and weight criteria. Once a patient is deemed to be a candidate for this type of procedure, 30–50 ml of autologous serum is prepared and frozen at −21 °C. The waiting time for a viable meniscal allograft averages 2 months—ranging from

R. Verdonk (✉)
Department of Orthopaedics and Trauma, University Hospital, De pintelaan 185,
9000 Ghent, Belgium
e-mail: Rene.verdonk@ugent.be

[1] Department of Orthopaedics and Trauma, Monica Ziekenhuizen, 2000 Antwerpen, Belgium.
[2] Department of Orthopaedics and Trauma, University Hospital, De pintelaan 185, 9000 Ghent, Belgium. e-mail: Rene.verdonk@ugent.be

R. Verdonk et al. (eds.), *Meniscal Transplantation*,
DOI: 10.1007/978-3-642-38106-5_4, © ISAKOS 2013

14 days to 6 months—at our institution. Once an appropriately sized meniscal allograft is harvested, the patient is notified and an operation is planned within the next 14 days.

4.1.2 Surgical Technique

4.1.2.1 Introduction

The purpose of this technical chapter is to present medial and lateral meniscal allograft transplantation (1) as an open procedure or (2) as an arthroscopically assisted procedure. Both techniques use primarily soft tissue fixation of the allograft to the native meniscal rim. Additional transosseus fixation of the anterior and posterior horn is used in the arthroscopic technique, while a tag on the anterior horn is used in the open procedure for soft tissue-bone fixation.

4.1.2.2 Anaesthesia and Surgical Preparation

These items are identical for the open and arthroscopic procedure.

The choice of anaesthesia is made in consultation between the surgeon, the anaesthesiologist and the patient and depends on patient's age, comorbidity and history with regard to previous anaesthesia. General anaesthesia is preferred at our institution.

The patient is then positioned supine on the operating table. A lateral leg-holder is positioned at the height of the tourniquet with the leg positioned in 90° of flexion. A foot holder is used to hold the leg in 90 and 110° of flexion as needed. Previous skin incisions are marked. The limb is exsanguinated and the tourniquet is inflated. The limb is then prepared with chlorhexidine gluconate-alcohol solution (Hibitane, Regent Medical Overseas Limited, Manchester, UK) and draped at the mid-thigh level.

4.1.2.3 Allograft Preparation for the Open Procedure

As previously described elsewhere, the allograft is positioned and fixed on a specially designed cork board with three 25 gauge needles [1]. With a scalpel, the residual synovial tissue is dissected from the allograft meniscus at the menisco-synovial junction level and discarded.

The upper side of the allograft is marked with a methylene blue skin marker.

Horizontal 2/0 polydioxanone surgical sutures (PDS II mounted on a double small needle, Ethicon, Somerville, NJ, USA) or 2/0 non-absorbable polypropylene sutures (Prolene mounted on a double small needle, Ethicon, Somerville, NJ, USA) are placed every 3–5 mm through the posterior horn, the body and the anterior horn of the allograft and fixed onto a specially designed suture holder (holder A). The senior surgeon (RV) prefers the use of 2/0 Prolene sutures for the posterior horn since this suture material comes with slightly smaller needles and therefore has easier surgical handling in the more narrow posterior joint space. The sutures are fixed onto the suture holder in sequence from posteriorly to anteriorly. Generally 6–8 sutures are needed to cover the complete allograft.

4.1.2.4 Open Meniscal Allograft Transplantation

A medial or lateral parapatellar incision of approximately 8 cm is made with the knee in 90° of flexion to gain access to the involved compartment of the knee joint. The joint capsule is then opened and the anterior horn of the meniscus remnant is transected.

For the lateral procedure, the iliotibial band is released subperiosteally from its distal attachment. To further open up the lateral compartment, the insertion the lateral collateral ligament (LCL) and popliteus tendon (PT) are detached with a curved osteotomy on the femoral side (Fig. 4.1). The centre of the osteotomy bone block is first predrilled with a 2.7 mm drill. This facilitates subsequent refixation with a screw and washer. The osteotomy is done in a clockwise direction from the 8 o'clock position to the 4 o'clock position and is approximately 1.5 cm deep and conically shaped. The bone block is gently folded out using a bone clamp and then the osteotomy is completed inferiorly from the 4 o'clock to the 8 o'clock position using the osteotome. The lateral joint space can now be opened up easily 1–2 cm by placing the knee in the figure of 4 position in 70–90° of flexion with the index foot positioned across the contralateral limb.

For the medial procedure, the medial collateral ligament is detached on the femoral side with an osteotomy [2]. A flake osteotomy (0.5–1 cm in thickness) is done with a straight osteotome at the level of the medial femoral epicondyle. The soft tissues posterior to the medial collateral ligament are left in continuity. By gently placing the knee in a valgus position, the medial compartment can now be opened up in a controlled fashion.

The meniscus remnant is trimmed preferably to a stable meniscal rim with a scalpel anteriorly and with arthroscopic instruments posteriorly. Most often, the insertion of the posterior horn is still intact and in continuity with the tibial plateau. The insertion of the posterior horn is also trimmed to fit the allograft. The meniscal

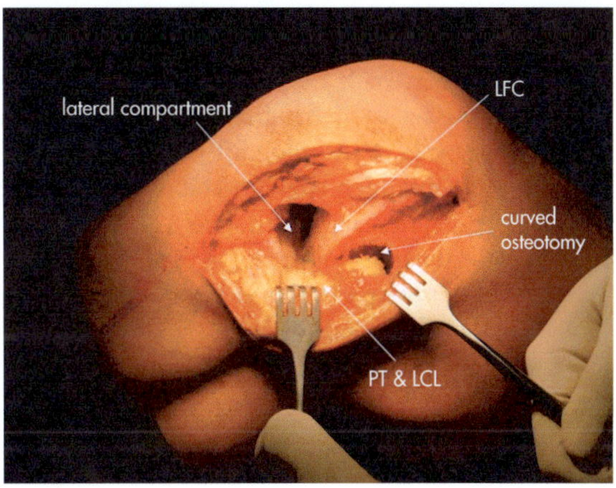

Fig. 4.1 Open meniscal allograft transplantation. To further open the lateral compartment, the LCL and PT are detached with a curved osteotomy on the femoral side

rim deserves surgical attention, as it serves as a strong envelope encapsulating the medial or lateral compartment of the knee.

The meniscal remnant level is then marked with a small mosquito clamp anteriorly as landmark for the correct level of subsequent fixation of the allograft. Next, the previously prepared viable meniscal allograft is introduced into the knee compartment. The sutures are taken from the holder in the correct sequence from posteriorly to anteriorly and driven through the meniscal rim one by one in an all-inside fashion from inferiorly to superiorly and transferred to a second suture holder (holder B), again in a sequence from posteriorly to anteriorly. The lateral allograft is also sutured to the popliteus tendon. We have found on follow-up arthroscopies that the popliteal hiatus will recreate itself naturally. The insertion of the anterior horn of the meniscus is not yet sutured at this stage of the operation. Once the sequence of suture transfer from holder A through the meniscal rim (and popliteal tendon) to holder B is completed, the allograft is introduced into the compartment by gently pulling on each suture in a sequence from posteriorly to anteriorly. Generally, this procedure has to be performed progressively to establish a secure fit of the allograft to the meniscal rim. The suture knots are then securely tied and cut. A fine-tipped suture driver and knot pusher are frequently required to securely tighten the posterior sutures. The knee is now positioned again in a normal 90° flexed position. The bone block of the collateral ligament and popliteus tendon is repositioned and fixed using a 35 or 40 mm 2.9 AO cancellous screw with a spiked washer. The anterior horn of the allograft is then fixed to the tibia using an anchor (GII, Depuy Mitek, Raynham, Massachussetts, USA). The Hoffa fat pad and knee capsule are closed using interrupted Vicryl 1/0 (Ethicon, Somerville, NJ, USA) cross stitches after haemostasis.

4.2 Arthroscopic Technique Without Bone Plugs

P. Verdonk[1]
R. Verdonk[2]

The allograft is positioned and fixed on a specially designed cork board with three 25 gauge needles. With a scalpel, the residual synovial tissue is dissected from the allograft meniscus at the meniscosynovial junction level and discarded.

The upper side of the allograft is marked with a methylene blue skin marker.

Non-resorbable high-strength (Fibre wire, Arthrex, Naples, USA) sutures are placed in the anterior and posterior horn of the allograft. Generally, 3 whipstitches are placed on the inner and outer rim of the horn of the allograft. An additional vertical non-resorbable suture (Ethibond 2/0, Somerville, NJ, USA) is placed at the posteromedial or posterolateral corner of the medial or lateral allograft, respectively. For the lateral allograft, the posterolateral suture is positioned just anteriorly to the popliteus tendon hiatus as this will serve as a landmark during arthroscopy (Fig. 4.2).

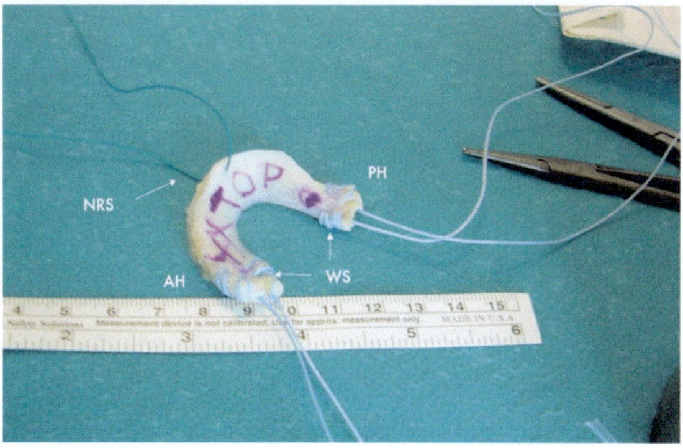

Fig. 4.2 Prepared lateral meniscal allograft for arthroscopic meniscal transplantation. Whipstiches (*WS*) on inner an outer rim of anterior (*AH*) and posterior horn (*PH*). A vertical non-resorbable suture (*NRS*) is placed on the posterolateral corner, just anteriorly of the PT hiatus

4.2.1 Arthroscopically Assisted Lateral Meniscal Allograft Transplantation

The classic anteromedial and anterolateral portals are made. An additional anteromedial portal is positioned very medially to gain easy instrumental access for the debridement and resection of the anterior portion of the native lateral meniscus. Using shaver and punch the remnant meniscus is debrided to the level of the meniscal rim.

A modified ACL aiming device, with a low profile tip, is inserted through the medial portal and positioned at the anatomical posterior horn of the lateral meniscus just posterior to the ACL (Fig. 4.3). A guide pin is drilled first and subsequently overdrilled by a 4.5 mm cannulated drill. A double loop metal wire is introduced through the tunnel from outside-in and picked up intra-articularly with an arthroscopical grasper and pulled out through the lateral portal. Subsequently, a suture passer (Acupass, Smith and Nephew, Memphis, Tennessee, USA) is introduced twice from outside-in just anterior to the lateral collateral ligament and

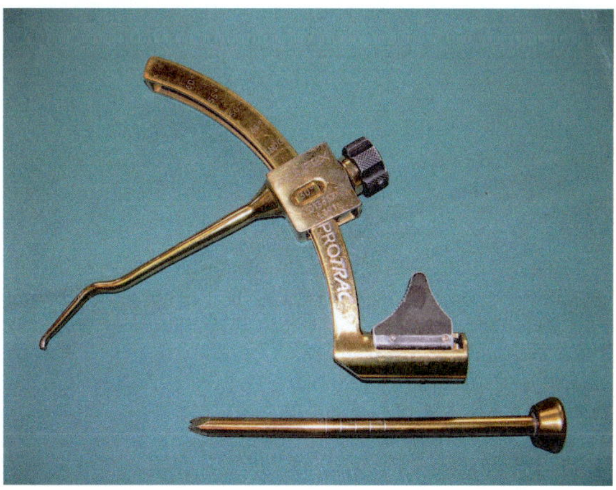

Fig. 4.3 Modified ACL aiming device, with low profile tip. This device is positioned at the anatomical posterior horn of the lateral meniscus, just posterior to the ACL

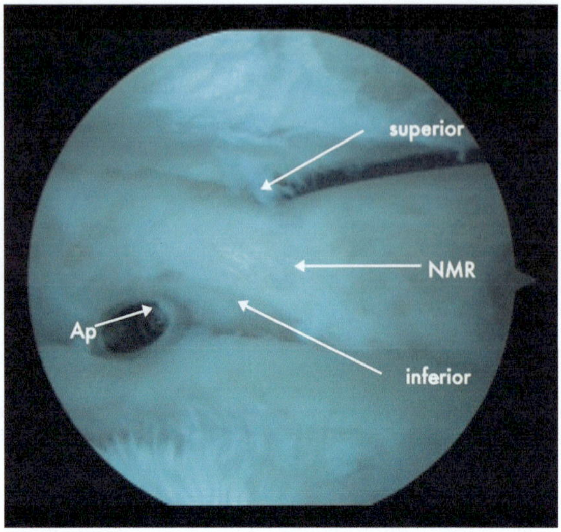

Fig. 4.4 A suture passer (Acupass®Ap) is introduced twice from outside-in, just anterior to the LCL and the PT, superior and inferior of the native meniscal rim (*NMR*)

the popliteus tendon into the joint: one just below and the second above the native meniscal rim (Fig. 4.4). The looped wires are picked up and pulled out again through the lateral portal. Next, the posterior horn pull suture and the posterolateral pull suture are pulled through using the double looped metal wire and the double looped suture pass wire. The prepared lateral allograft is subsequently introduced into the lateral compartment throughout an enlarged lateral portal by pulling progressively on the posterolateral pull suture and the posterior horn pull suture. Care should be taken that the graft does not flip upon introduction and that pull wires do not intertwine. Risk for intertwining wires is greatly reduced by using a double loop metal wire for the posterior horn.

The posterior horn is now positioned correctly. Its position can be slightly modified more towards the posterolateral corner or more towards the posterior horn by pulling more on the posterolateral or posterior horn traction wire. One or two all-inside meniscal fixation devices (Fastfix, Smith and Nephew, Memphis, Tennessee, USA) are used to fix the allograft to the meniscal rim. Fixation should be started in the posterolateral corner. Subsequently inside out horizontal Ethibond 2/0 sutures are used for fixing the body of the allograft. The anterior horn is fixed using outside in PDS or Ethibond 2/0 sutures.

Prior to making the sutures knots, the anterior horn is introduced into the knee joint and the anatomical insertion site is identified and prepared is a same manner as for the posterior tunnel. If necessary, its position can be slightly adapted to the graft position. Similar to the procedure of the posterior horn, the anterior tunnel is prepared and the traction suture is pulled through.

First, the meniscal inside out sutures are knotted. Subsequently, the anterior and posterior horn traction sutures are knotted to each other over a bone bridge on the anteromedial side of the tibia. This procedure reduces the possibly stretched capsule and native meniscal rim tied to the meniscal allograft, by pulling on the anterior and posterior horn by a transosseus suture fixation.

4.2.2 Arthroscopically Assisted Medial Meniscal Allograft Transplantation

A similar procedure as for the lateral allograft transplantation is performed for the medial allograft transplantation. However, some steps are different and will be highlighted in this section.

Additional to the classic anteromedial and anterolateral portal, a posteromedial portal should be used to identify the original posterior horn attachments of the native meniscus (Fig. 4.5). Using the same drill guide, the transosseus tunnels can be prepared. These tunnels should be prepared starting on the anterolateral side of the tibia. This direction is more in line with the forces on the traction sutures.

A posteromedial traction suture is used, as in accordance to the lateral allograft. On the medial side, however, we lack a clear anatomical landmark such as the popliteal hiatus on the lateral side.

The anterior horn of the native medial meniscus may in some cases be very anterior on the tibial plateau resulting in a very short transosseus anterior tunnel.

4.2.2.1 Special Note on Soft Tissue Versus Bone Block Fixation [3–7]

Biomechanical cadaver studies have shown the superiority of a bony fixation over a soft tissue fixation technique, although a recent cadaver study showed comparable results. Bony fixation however, has also been shown to be associated with increased risk for cartilage lesions if implanted incorrectly and an increased

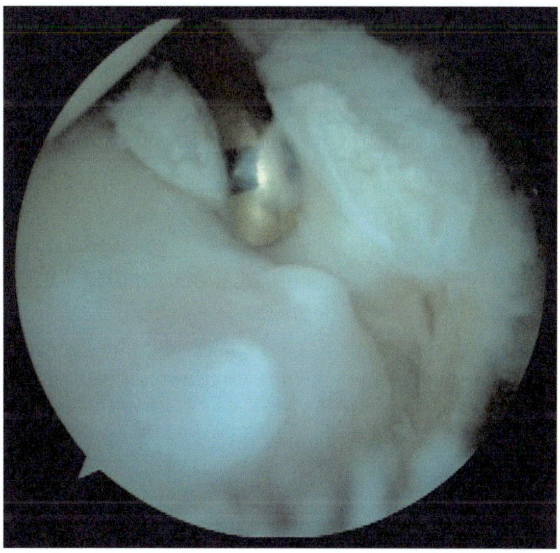

Fig. 4.5 Arthroscopical view of the posteromedial portal used in arthroscopically assisted medial meniscal allograft transplantation. The custum ACL guide in introduced through the intercondylar notch on the anatomical posterior horn insertion of the native medial meniscus

immunological potential due to the presence of allogeneic bone. It is the authors experience that perfect allograft size matching is essential if bony fixation is to be used. A malpositioned bone block or plugs can inflict damages to the overlying cartilage. Too small a graft will result in a need to overtension the inside out sutures and possible failure of the soft tissue fixation. Therefore, limited oversizing of the graft is commonly advocated using bone plugs or blocks. Separate bone plugs have the potential advantage that the implantation can be somewhat more variable compared to a single bone block. In addition, on the lateral side a straight bone block sometimes induces the need to sacrifice some posterolateral fibers of the ACL.

Today, clinical and/or radiological differences have not been shown between soft tissue or bone block fixation.

4.2.3 Rehabilitation

Rehabilitation is initially focused on providing mobility to the joint without endangering ingrowth and healing of the graft. Therefore, 3 weeks of non-weight-bearing are prescribed followed by 3 weeks of partial weight bearing (50 % of body weight). Progression to full weight bearing is allowed from week 6 on to week 10 postoperatively. The use of a knee brace is not strictly necessary and depends on the morphology and profile of the patient. For the same reasons, range of motion is limited during the first 2 weeks from 0 to 30, to increase by 30° each 2 weeks.

Isometric muscle tonification and co-contraction exercises are prescribed from day 1 post-surgery on. Straight leg raise however, is prohibited during the first 3 weeks. Proprioception training is started after week 3.

Swimming is allowed after week 6, biking after week 12 and running is progressively promoted starting at week 20.

4.3 Conclusion

In conclusion, ample evidence has been presented to support meniscus allograft transplantation in meniscectomized painful knees, with observance of the proper indications. Significant relief of pain and improvement in function have been achieved in a high percentage of patients. These improvements appear to be long-lasting in 70 % of patients. Based on plain radiology and MRI, a subset of patients does not show further cartilage degeneration, indicating a potential chondro-protective effect. The lack of a conservatively treated control group is considered a fundamental flaw in the reported studies, making it difficult to establish the true chondro-protective effect of this type of treatment. Based on the presented results, meniscus allograft transplantation should no longer be considered experimental surgery for the meniscectomized painful knee (Table 4.1).

Table 4.1 International cartilage repair society cartilage lesion evaluation system

Grade 0	Normal
Grade 1	Superficial lesions, softening, fissures or cracks
Grade 2	Lesions, erosion or ulceration of less than 50 %
Grade 3	Partial-thickness defect of more than 50 %, but less than 100 %
Grade 4	Ulceration and bone exposure

4.4 Arthroscopic Technique with Bone Plugs

P. E. Gelber[3]
H. Pereira[4]
J. Espregueira-Mendes[5]
J. C. Monllau[6]

The key objective of the AMT is the alleviation of knee pain and an improvement in knee function for patients that have been submitted to meniscectomy. The correct anatomic positioning and stable fixation of the graft are the main technical targets. Although it may be easier to secure the graft by managing soft tissue alone, cadaver model research indicates superior transmission of load occurs when the meniscal horns of the graft are fixed to the tibia [7].

Bony fixation can be achieved with bone plugs attached to the anterior and posterior horns or simply a bone bridge. The former allows a less invasive technique and might preserve the tibial eminence. There is great variability in medial meniscus anterior horn insertion types and these variants must be respected when replacing the original meniscus [8]. This can be better achieved with bone tunnels but not with the use of a bone bridge. However, it is technically highly demanding due to the fact that minimal misplacement of the tibial tunnels may lead to improper functioning of the meniscal graft [9]. The bone bridge technique better preserves the native distance between horns and eliminates the risk of their incorrect placement. It is particularly useful in lateral meniscus transplantation as the insertions of the lateral meniscus are quite close and there is less variability.

[3] Department of Orthopaedic Surgery, Hospital de la Sta Creu i Sant Pau, ICATME- Institut Universitari Dexeus, Universitat Autònoma de Barcelona, St AM Claret, 167, 08025 Barcelona, Spain. e-mail: Pgelber@santpau.cat

[4] Clínica Espregueira-Mendes, Estádio do Dragão, 4350-415 Porto, Portugal. e-mail: heldermdpereira@gmail.com

[5] Clínica Espregueira-Mendes, Estádio do Dragão, 4350-415 Porto, Portugal. e-mail: jem@espregueira.com,

[6] Department of Orthopaedic Surgery, Hospital de la Sta Creu i Sant Pau, ICATME- Institut Universitari Dexeus, Universitat Autònoma de Barcelona, St AM Claret, 167, 08025 Barcelona, Spain. e-mail: Jmonllau@santpau.cat

However, it is a more invasive technique because it affects tibial eminence integrity and resects more bone.

While medial meniscus transplantation is more commonly performed with bone plugs, most authors advocate performing AMT in the lateral meniscus with the bone bridge technique. It is more appropriate as the distance between the horns of the lateral meniscus is typically less than 1 cm. Therefore, tibial tunnel collision and a consequent compromised fixation of the horns might result if a bone-plug technique is used. The medial meniscus can also be transplanted with a bone bridge technique, but this requires careful placement so as not to alter the ACL tibial insertion. Furthermore, interference between bone trough and tibial tunnel may occur if an ACL reconstruction is to be associated at the same time.

The authors advocate the use of bone plugs in the medial meniscus transplantation and bone bridge for the lateral one.

4.4.1 Patient Positioning

A thigh tourniquet, inflated after the sterile field is prepared, is recommended. Alternatively, the use of a pump is also a good option as it keeps the joint clean allowing for a good vision without time limitation. Positioning depends mainly of surgeon's experience and comfort. Placing the patient supine was found to be easier for the authors. In the case of a medial AMT, both legs are left hanging free at 90° flexion. The use of a thigh lateral post permits applying valgus stress to open-up the medial compartment. If a lateral AMT is to be done, the contralateral limb is placed in extension. It allows for the figure-of-four-position without the help of an assistant.

4.4.2 Graft Preparation

Medial AMT: After thawing in saline solution with antibiotic at room temperature, the residual synovial tissue from the graft is dissected at the meniscosinovial junction in order to facilitate graft introduction into the joint and suture technique.

A 1.0 mm Kirschner wire is drilled through the centre of the horn attachments prior to bone plug preparation. The hole will be used to pass the traction sutures, and placing first the kirschner wire will facilitate harvesting the plug without the hole collapsing. Bone plugs of 5–6 mm of diameter and 8–10 mm of height, including the anatomic meniscal attachments to the tibia, are then prepared. Both horns are sutured in a whipstitch manner and the suture also includes the bone plugs (through the previously drilled hole) thus making the graft insertion into the joint as well as accommodation of the bone plugs in the prepared bone tunnels easier (Fig. 4.6a and b).

The upper side of the meniscus as well as the union between the middle and posterior thirds are marked with a skin marker. This will help in avoiding improper placement of the graft during insertion. A third traction suture is placed at the

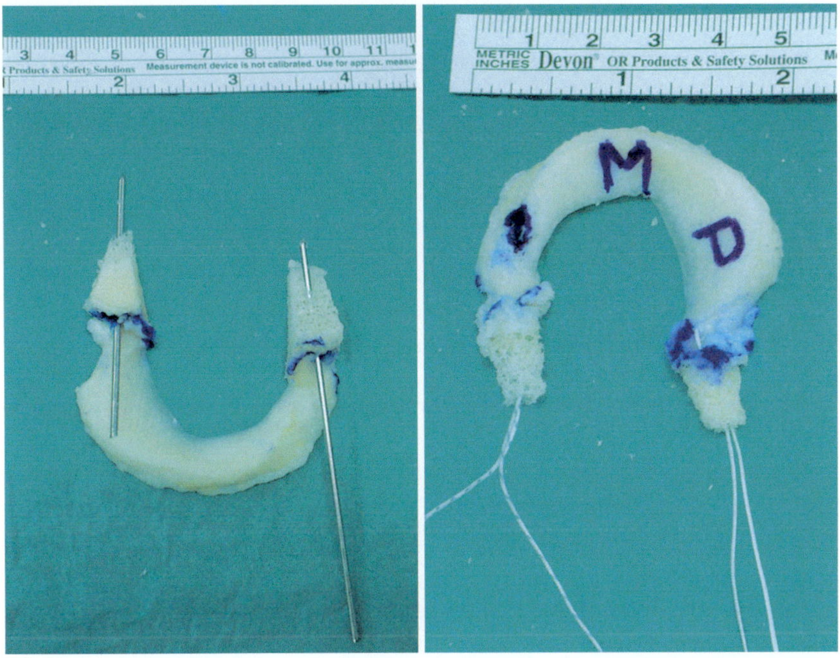

Fig. 4.6 Medial meniscal graft preparation. Note the k-wires passing through the bone plugs

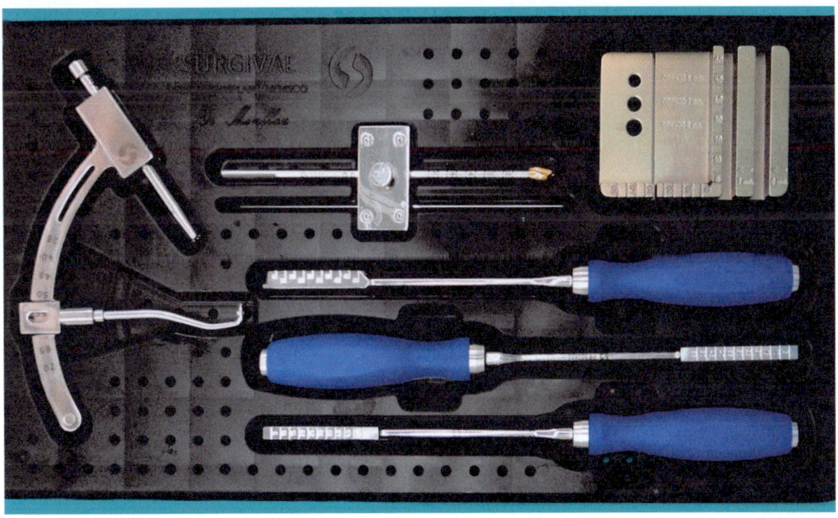

Fig. 4.7 Surgical meniscal transplant set of instruments

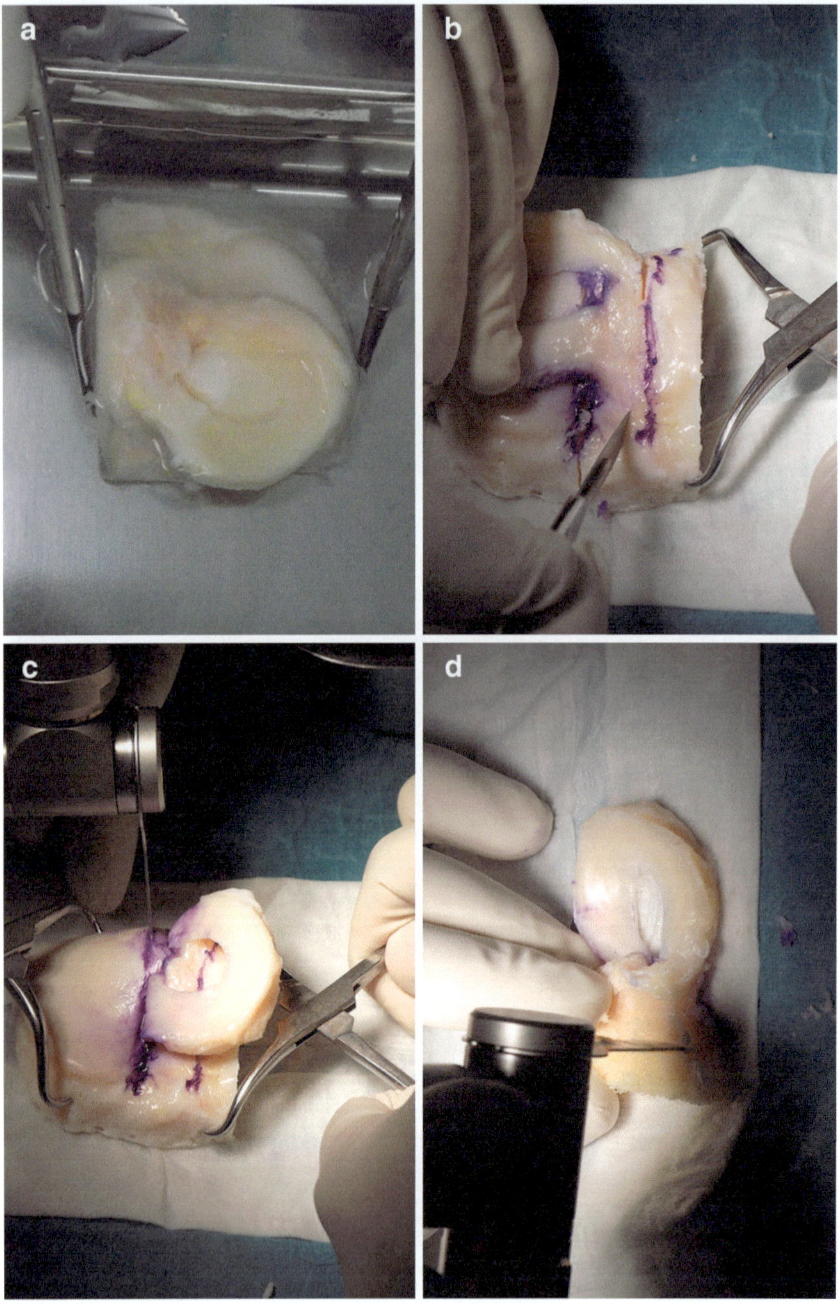

Fig. 4.8 **a**, **b**, **c** and **d** showing the preparation of a lateral meniscus graft for the bridge and slot technique

junction between the posterior horn and the body of the meniscus where the pencil mark had been made. This will greatly help in placing the posterior horn of the prepared graft into the posterior aspect of the joint.

Once the AMT is harvested, it is wrapped with a wet gauze soak in a saline solution with antibiotic until introduced into the receptor knee.

Lateral AMT: After thawing and dissecting any residual tissue, the hemiplateau with its meniscus on top is brought to the work station (Meniscal Transplantion Set. Surgival. Paterna. Spain) (Fig. 4.7). A bone bridge from anterior to posterior horn of 7–8 mm width and 10 mm high is drawn with a pen and harvested with the aid of a small saw and a chisel (Fig. 4.8a, b, c, d). Since the bone bridge gives optimal stability, no predrilled tibial tunnel or additional traction sutures on the bone block are needed (Fig. 4.9).

A traction suture at the middle and posterior thirds of the graft and upper side marks will be prepared as described for the medial allograft. Once harvested, the graft is also embedded in a gauze soak in saline solution with antibiotic until introduced into the receptor knee.

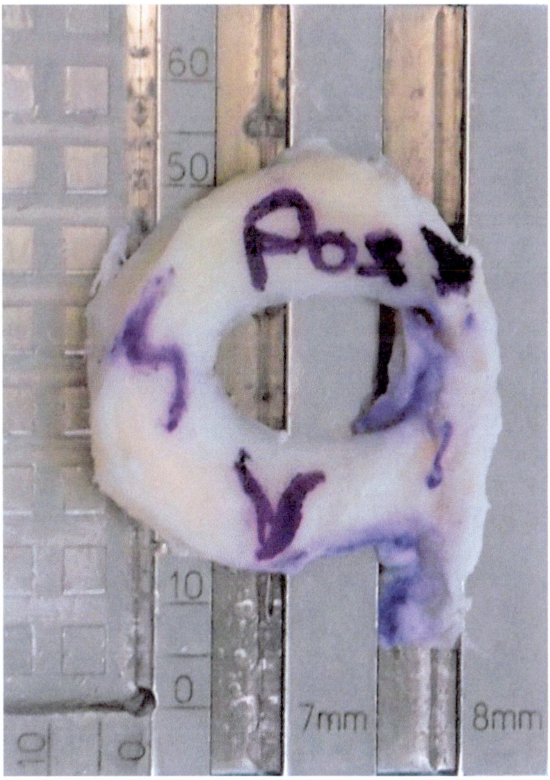

Fig. 4.9 The lateral meniscus graft once prepared and conveniently marked and sized utilizing a metal cutting block

4.4.3 Arthroscopic Procedure

A routine diagnostic arthroscopy is done through a standard anterolateral viewing portal. Medial portal and additional accessory portals are established depending on the compartment to be transplanted. The remaining meniscus is debrided to get a stable rim and guarantee a good blood supply. It is important not to eliminate the entire meniscal rim as it may help the suturing and limit later allograft extrusion by maintaining meniscus hoop stress. For that purpose, the authors recommend limiting mechanical debridement by using high frequency or radiofrequency trephination. Radiofrequency creates an area of synovial necrosis adjacent to the graft that is promptly substituted by a newly formed and more vascular synovial

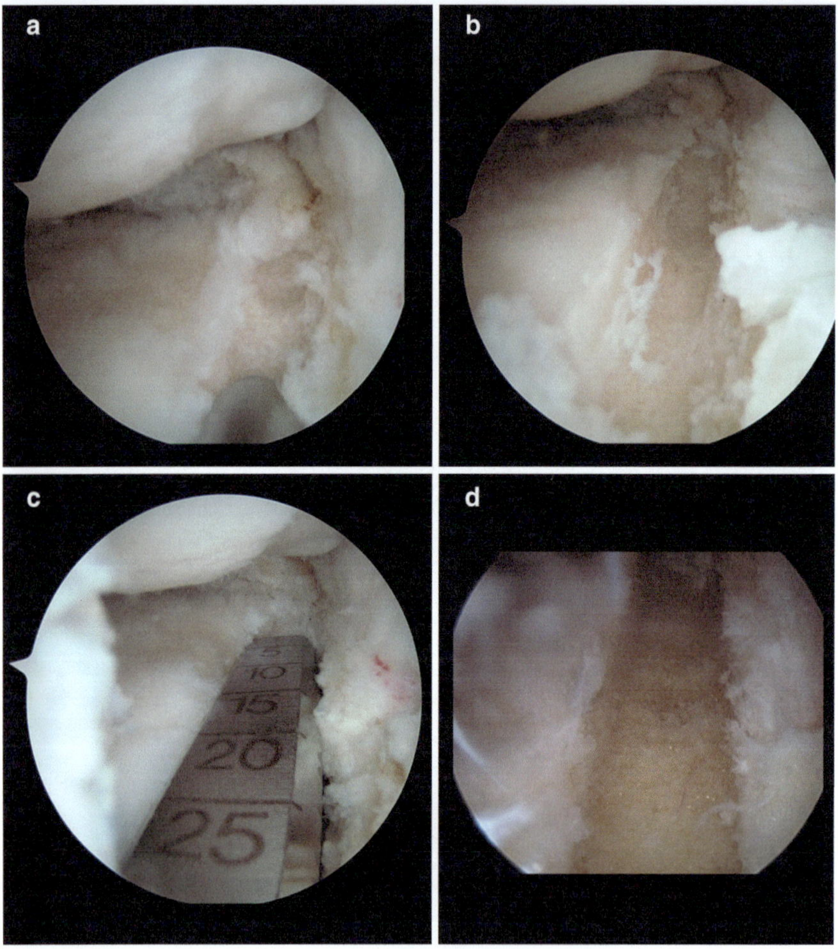

Fig. 4.10 Arthroscopic view of the lateral compartment. Using a burr **a** followed by a drill, **b** and a set of rasps, **c** a completely quadrangle trough, **d** is created

layer that invades the allograft as a wave and retires over time thus creating an appropriate nutritional supply to the graft [10, 11].

A prominent tibial spine might prevent the correct visualization of the medial meniscus posterior horn. Under that circumstance, the tibial spine can be flattened with a burr, thus leaving room enough to introduce the scope or a tibial guide [12].

4.4.4 Bone Fixation

If a bone plug technique is to be used, exact positioning of the tibial tunnels for both meniscal horns is mandatory. As well described by Kohn and Moreno, they must be placed at the anatomical insertion sites [13]. The tibial tunnels are drilled with the help of a standard or modified ACL tibial guide. The traction suture is placed at the union of the middle and posterior thirds of the remaining meniscus using an outside-in technique with two 18-gauge spinal needles. This suture is first retrieved from the posteromedial corner and will help with graft introduction into the joint and the posterior accommodation of its posterior horn. Meniscal horn sutures are passed through the corresponding tibial bone tunnels with the help of a suture passer. Then, the graft must be placed in its bed simply by enlarging the portal (minarthrotomy) and pulling the sutures. These maneuvers are important to making introduction of the graft easier. Traction from both meniscal horns and from the posteromedial traction suture will help to firmly attach the AMT in its

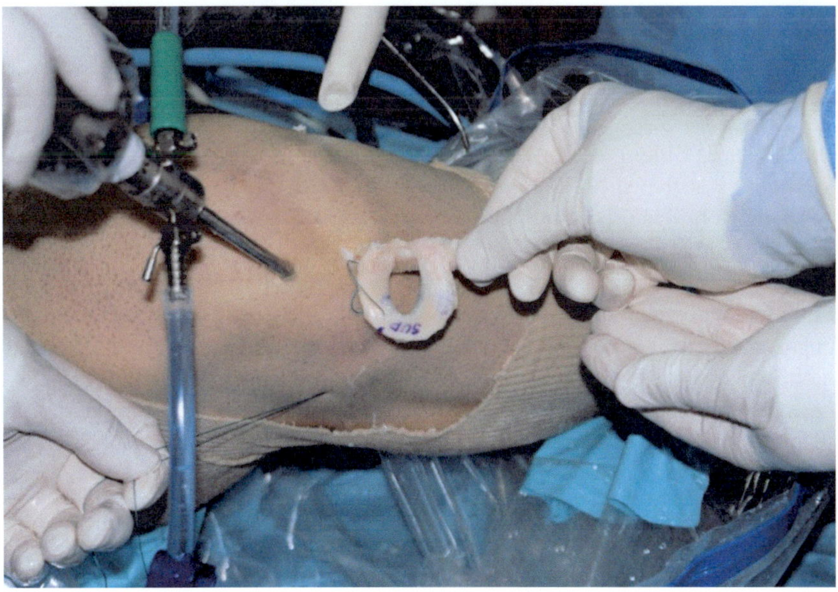

Fig. 4.11 The right knee in a figure of four position with a miniarthrotomy and a traction suture placed in the posterolateral corner to facilitate the introduction of the graft

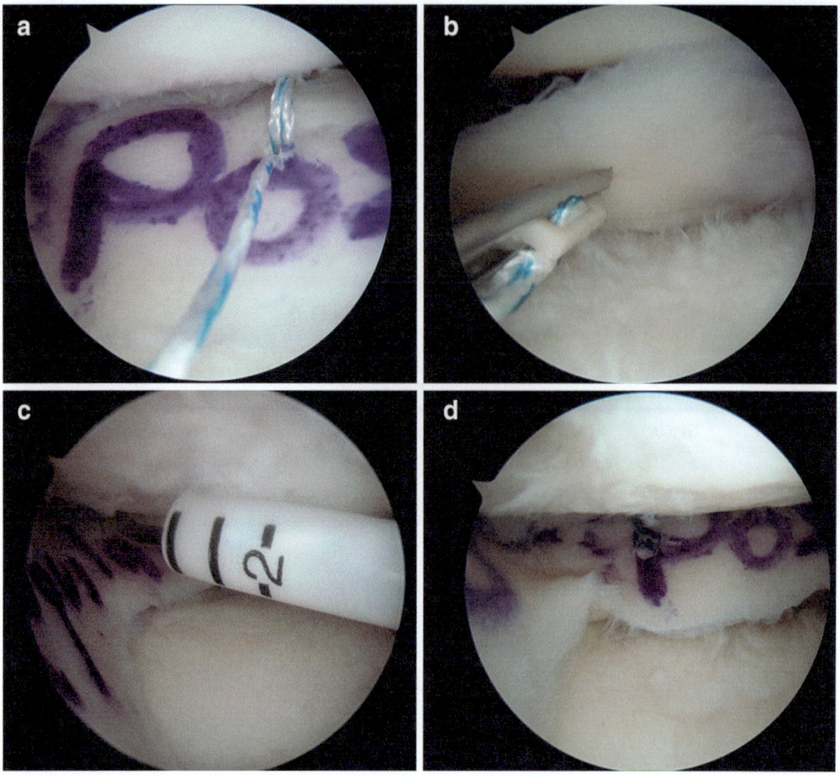

Fig. 4.12 All-inside suture combining vertical and horizontal mattress sutures alternatively placed in the upper and lower sides of a lateral meniscus graft

former place. Bone plugs are secured by tying the sutures to each other on the tibial cortex at the end of the procedure.

The bone bridge procedure requires the creation of a trough in the tibial plateau using the bridge-in-slot technique [14]. In this technique, a guide pin connecting the anterior and posterior horns is followed by a drill and finally shaped with a 7 or 8 mm width box cutter to simply create the trough (Fig. 4.10). The same width and length matched size must be obtained with the graft. The authors prefer to create the trough progressively by using a burr followed by a drill and a set of rasps. All these instruments are brought into the joint creating a lateral or medial portal just in line with the desired position of the planned trough. The so-called *keyhole* technique, which creates the cross-section of the bridge like a keyhole, can optionally be used. The graft must be placed in its bed simply by enlarging the portal some 3–4 cm (minarthrotomy) and sliding the bone block (Fig. 4.11). As already mentioned, the traction suture from the posterolateral corner will help to put the AMT in its place. The bone bar can be fixed with interference screws or left

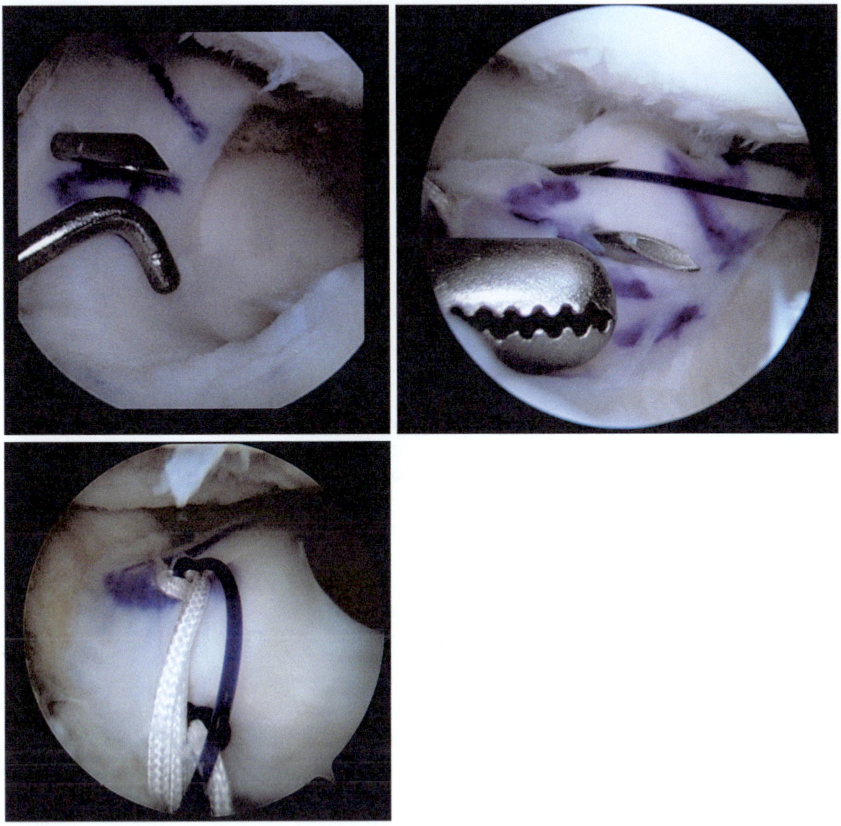

Fig. 4.13 Outside-in suturing of the anterior third of the graft

alone, as the authors do, assuming that the bar is kept in place by the joint congruence.

Finally, all-inside (FasT-Fix™ Suture System. Smith & Nephew, Inc., Andover, MA 01810, USA) or inside-out suturing, depending on the preferences of the surgeon, is performed at the posterior horn and body of the meniscus allograft (Fig. 4.12). If an inside-out suture technique is used, and additional posteromedial or posterolateral portal is necessary to retrieve sutures in a safe manner. The anterior horn can be better fixed with an outside-in technique using a couple of 18-gauge spinal needles (Fig. 4.13).

An intra-articular drain can optionally be used. Nevertheless, it is the authors' opinion that some residual blood in the joint might enhance the meniscal healing process. The lower limb is finally placed in an immobilizer with a simple dressing to make it easy to apply an ice-pack in the postoperative period.

References

1. Verdonk PC, Demurie A, Almqvist KF, Veys EM, Verbruggen G, Verdonk R (2006) Transplantation of viable meniscal allograft. Surgical technique. J Bone Joint Surg Am Mar 88:109–118. Review
2. Goble EM, Verdonk R, Kohn D (1999) Arthroscopic and open surgical techniques for meniscus replacement–meniscal allograft transplantation and tendon autograft transplantation. Scand J Med Sci Sports 9(3):168–176
3. Messner K, Verdonk R (1999) It is necessary to anchor the meniscal transplants with bone plugs? A mini-battle. Scand J Med Sci Sports 9(3):186–187
4. Paletta GA Jr, Manning T, Snell E, Parker R, Bergfeld J (1997) The effect of allograft meniscal replacement on intraarticular contact area and pressures in the human knee. A biomechanical study. Am J Sports Med 25:692–698
5. Huang A, Hull ML, Howell SM (2003) The level of compressive load affects conclusions from statistical analyses to determine whether a lateral meniscal autograft restores tibial contact pressure to normal: a study in human cadaveric knees. J Orthop Res 21:459–464
6. Chen MI, Branch TP, Hutton WC (1996) Is it important to secure the horns during lateral meniscal transplantation? A cadaveric study. Arthroscopy 12:174–181
7. Alhalki MM, Howell SM, Hull ML (1999) How three methods for fixing a medial meniscal autograft affect tibial contact mechanics. Am J Sports Med 27:320–328
8. Berlet GC, Fowler PJ (1998) The anterior horn of the medial meniscus: an anatomic study of its insertion. Am J Sports Med 26:540–543
9. Sekaran SV, Hull ML, Howell SM (2002) Nonanatomic location of the posterior horn of a medial meniscal autograft implanted in a cadaveric knee adversely affects the pressure distribution on the tibial plateau. Am J Sports Med 30:74–82
10. Iñigo-Pavlovich R (2005) Radiofrequency and meniscus. From excision to repair. Sports Med Arthrosc Rev 13:193–197
11. Monllau JC, Leal J, Voss C, Pelfort X, Tey M, Pavlovich RI (2010) Good outcome after meniscal repair using an all-inside suturing system in combination with high-frequency biostimulation. Orthopedics 33(6):407–412
12. Monllau JC, Gonzalez-Lucena G, Gelber P, Pelfort X (2010) Allograft meniscus transplantation: a current review. Tech Knee Surg 9(2):107–113
13. Kohn D, Moreno B (1995) Meniscus insertion anatomy as a basis for meniscus replacement: a morphological cadaveric study. Arthroscopy 11:96–103
14. Farr J, Meneghini RM, Cole BJ (2004) Allograft interference screw fixation in meniscus transplantation. Arthroscopy 20:322–327

Results and Indications

5

P. Verdonk and R. Verdonk

5.1 Indications and Contraindications

5.1.1 Indications

According to current recommendations, meniscal allograft transplantation is indicated in three specific clinical settings:

1. Young patients with a history of meniscectomy who have pain localized to the meniscus-deficient compartment, a stable knee joint, no malalignment, and articular cartilage with only minor evidence of osteochondral degenerative changes [no more than grade 3 according to the International Cartilage Repair Society (ICRS) classification system (Table 5.1)], are considered ideal candidates for this procedure. Some studies [1–6] have shown that meniscal allografts can survive in an osteoarthritic joint (Outerbridge grade 3–4), with significant improvement in pain and function. Because of the more rapid deterioration in the lateral compartment [7], a relatively common indication for meniscal transplantation would be a symptomatic, meniscus-deficient, lateral compartment.
2. Anterior cruciate ligament (ACL)-deficient patients who have had previous medial meniscectomy with concomitant ACL reconstruction and who might benefit from the increased stability afforded by a functional medial meniscus. It is the authors' conviction, that an ACL graft is significantly protected by the meniscus allograft as much as the meniscus is protected by an ACL graft.

P. Verdonk
Department of Orthopaedics and Trauma, Monica Ziekenhuizen, 2000, Antwerpen, Belgium

R. Verdonk (✉)
Department of Orthopaedics and Trauma, University Hospital, De pintelaan 185, 9000, Gent, Belgium
e-mail: Rene.verdonk@ugent.be

R. Verdonk et al. (eds.), *Meniscal Transplantation*,
DOI: 10.1007/978-3-642-38106-5_5, © ISAKOS 2013

Table 5.1 International cartilage repair society cartilage lesion evaluation system

Grade 0	Normal
Grade 1	Superficial lesions, softening, fissures or cracks
Grade 2	Lesions, erosion or ulceration of less than 50 %
Grade 3	Partial-thickness defect of more than 50 % but less than 100 %
Grade 4	Ulceration and bone exposure

3. In an effort to avert early joint degeneration, some also consider young, athletic patients who have had total meniscectomy, as candidates for meniscal transplantation prior to symptom onset [8]. *However, the results obtained so far still preclude a return to high-impact sports.*

5.1.2 Contraindications

Advanced chondral degeneration is considered a contraindication to meniscal allograft transplantation, although some studies suggest that cartilage degeneration is not a significant risk factor for failure [9]. In general, greater than grade 3 articular cartilage lesions according to the ICRS classification system should be of limited surface area and localized. Localized chondral defects may be treated concomitantly, as meniscus transplantation and cartilage repair or restoration may benefit each other in terms of healing and outcome [10]. Chondrocyte transplantation or osteochondral grafting procedures should be performed after completion of the meniscal transplantation in order to prevent accidental damage to the patch or graft during meniscal allograft insertion [11]. Radiographic evidence of significant osteophyte formation or femoral condyle flattening is associated with inferior postoperative results because these structural modifications alter the morphology of the femoral condyle [12]. Generally, patients over age 50 have excessive cartilage lesions and are suboptimal candidates.

Axial malalignment tends to exert abnormal pressure on the allograft leading to loosening, degeneration, and failure of the graft [12]. A corrective osteotomy should be considered in patients with more than two degrees of deviation toward the involved compartment, as compared with the mechanical axis of the contralateral limb. Varus or valgus deformity may be managed with either staged or concomitant high tibial or distal femoral osteotomy [11]. However, as in any situation in which procedures are combined, it is unclear which aspect of the procedure is implicated in symptom resolution, such as relief of pain [12].

Other contraindications to meniscal transplantation are obesity, skeletal immaturity, instability of the knee joint (which may be addressed in conjunction with transplantation), synovial disease, inflammatory arthritis and previous joint infection, and obvious squaring of the femoral condyle.

5.2 Results

It is difficult to perform a meta-analysis of all the published results, because of the small populations studied and the differences (Table 5.2) in indications, contra-indications, preservation techniques, preoperative Outerbridge grade, fixation techniques, surgical techniques, concomitant procedures, evaluation tools and rehabilitation protocols.

In this chapter, we will try to present outcome data based on a review of the literature. A total of 39 studies have been included, representing 1,226 meniscus allografts (626 medial vs. 446 lateral, 154 not specified) in 1,145 patients. The mean age at the time of surgery was 34.4 years. The mean follow-up was 5.5 years. Overall, 340 isolated allograft transplantations were analysed, 427 were associated with ACL reconstruction, 107 with a corrective osteotomy and 215 with other procedures. It was not specified whether the remaining 137 allografts were associated with other procedures. Concerning the surgical fixation technique, 631 allografts were fixed using bone blocks and 488 using a soft-tissue fixation technique. For 107 allografts the fixation method was not specified. In the next paragraphs, the outcome is reported independently of the aforementioned parameters.

Methods to evaluate the success or failure of meniscal transplantation range from subjective pain scale measurements and patient perceptions of function to objective measurements such as physical and radiological examinations, magnetic resonance imaging (MRI), and second-look arthroscopy.

5.2.1 Subjective Assessment

All studies showed significant subjective improvement in pain scales and functional activity questionnaires. The data from most studies are summarized in Table 5.3. In general, isolated procedures and combined procedures tended to have similar outcomes. No differences were observed based on tissue preservation technique or fixation method. About 75–90 % of patients experienced fair to excellent results.

5.2.2 Objective Clinical Scoring

5.2.2.1 Physical Examination

Almost all studies reported equal or improved physical examination findings at follow-up with regard to range of motion, pain, effusion, stability, function tests or IKDC score. The data from most studies are summarized in Table 5.4.

Table 5.2 The difficulty realizing a meta analysis of all the published results, because of the small populations studied and the differences in indications, contraindications, preservation techniques, preoperative outerbridge grade, fixation techniques, surgical techniques, concomitant procedures, evaluation tools and rehabilitation protocols

Nr	Authors	Year P	Year S	# grafts	M	L	# patients	Age	Time M-TX	Preservation	Rad?	Fix	FUT	Preop cart	# isolated	Concomm. procedures
1.	Cameron and Saha.	1997	1988–1994	67	37	30	63	41	16.7	DF	Yes	S	2.5	2–4	21	5ACL, 34OT, 7ACL+OT
2.	Carter et al.	1999	NA	46	39	7	46	NA	NA	Cryo.	NA	B	2.8	NA	NA	30ACL, 4OT, 1MCL
3.	Garrett et al.	1993	NA	43	34	8	43	NA	NA	16DF, 27Cryo.	NA	B	4.5	NA	7	24ACL, 13OT, 11OAL
4.	Goble et al.	1999	NA	69	48	21	60	NA	NA	Cryo.	NA	B	2	NA	NA	28ACL
5.	Groff et al.	2001	1993–1998	16	0	16	16	27	8	DF	No	B	3.8	1–2	16	None
6.	Wirth et al.	2002	1984–1986	22	22	0	22	29.6	NA	6DF, 16Lyo.	6No, 16Yes	S	3/14	1, 6	0	22ACL, 19MCL
7.	Noyes et al.	1995	NA	96	79	17	83	NA	NA	DF	Yes	B	<2	NA	19	77ACL
8.		2004	1995–2000	40	20	20	38	30	NA	Cryo.	No	B	3.3	3, 6	NA	7ACL, 1PCL, 1ACL+PCL, 1MCL, 16 OAU
9.	Rath et al.	2001	1991–1997	22	15	7	18	30	7.7	Cryo. + DF	No	1S, 21B	4.5	NA	3	11ACL, 1TTT
10.	Stollsteimer et al.	2000	1991–1995	23	11	12	22	31	3.8	Cryo.	No	B	3.3	COB: 5, 6	23	None
11.	Van Arkel et al.	2000	1994–1995	19	6	13	16	40	16	Cryo.	No	NA	2.7	NA	NA	NA
12.		2002	1989–1999	63	23	40	57	39	16	Cryo.	No	S	5	NA	61	2ACL
13.	Verdonk et al.	2004	NA	27	0	27	27	33,9	NA	V	No	S	1	NA	NA	NA
14.		2005	1989–2001	100	39	61	96	35	NA	V	No	S	7.2	2.5	69	3ACL, 17OT, 3Mi, 4OPT
15.		2006	1989–1993	39	NA	NA	38	35.4	NA	V	No	S	12.1	2.7	NA	3ACL, 12OT

(continued)

Table 5.2 (continued)

Nr	Authors	Year P	Year S	# grafts	M	L	# patients	Age	Time M-TX	Preservation	Rad?	Fix	FUT	Preop cart	# isolated	Concomm. procedures
16.	Shelton and Dukes	1994	NA	14	5	9	14	NA	NA	Cryo.	NA	B	NA	NA	NA	NA
17.	Veltri et al.	1994	NA	16	8	8	14	35,3	11,3	DF + Cryo.	No	B	0.7	NA	4	10ACL, 1PCL, 1ACL+PCL
18.	Cole et al.	2006	1997–2003	40	25	15	36	31	NA	32DF + 8Cryo.	No	B	2.8	<4	21	ACL, 1OT, 3OAL, 3OAU, 1ACI, 2Mi, 2 ODfix
19.	Rodeo et al.	2000	1989–1995	33	17	16	28	34	NA	DF	No	20B, 13S	1.3	NA	8	19ACL, 1OT
20.	Del Pizzo et al.	1996	1991–1994	19	NA	NA	19	NA	NA	19Cryo.	NA	NA	3.2	NA	6	11ACL, 2OT
21.	Yoldas et al.	2003	1993–1996	34	NA	NA	31	28	8	DF	No	B	2.9	NA	11	20ACL
22.	Ryu et al.	2002	1993–1999	26	10	16	25	34.5	NA	NA	NA	B	2.75	2.8	12	14ACL
23.	Hommen et al.	2007	1991–1995	20	12	8	20	32	NA	20Cryo.	No	13S, 7B	11.7	2.2	5	10ACL, 2OT, 3CHFC, 2CP, 3LR
24.	Cryolife	1997	1989–1994	1023	747	276	1015	NA	NA	Cryo.	NA	930B, 92S	7	NA	NA	NA
25.	Felix and Paulos	2002	1993–1999	36	20	16	33	28.5	6	Cryo.	No	B	5.2	NA	9	18ACL, 2OT, 4ACL+OT
26.	Vacquero et al.	2003	2001–2002	32	NA	NA	30	37	NA	DF	No	B	>1	2, 3	NA	6ACL, 3Mi, 7RFA, 1TTT
27.	Sekiya et al.	2003	1994–1998	31	24	7	28	35	8.6	Cryo.	No	B	2.8	1–4	0	28ACL, 2ACL+OT
28.		2006	1993–1998	25	0	25	25	30	5.7	Cryo.	No	8S, 17B	3.3	1–4	25	None

(continued)

Table 5.2 (continued)

Nr	Authors	Year P	Year S	# grafts	M	L	# patients	Age	Time M-TX	Preservation	Rad?	Fix	FUT	Preop cart	# isolated	Concomm. procedures
29.	Potter et al.	1996	1989–1996	29	14	15	24	33.2	NA	DF	NA	B	NA	2–4	11	16ACL, 1OT, 1MCL
30.	Stone et al.	2006	1997–1999	47	37	10	45	48	NA	18DF, 29Cryo.	No	S	5.8	3.8	7	6ACL, 17OT, 19Mi, 47CHFC, 24ACPG
31.	Fukushima et al.	2004	1996–1997	43	30	13	40	37.3	11.4	Cryo.	No	S	1	NA	NA	8ACL, 1OT
32.	Rankin et al.	2006	NA	8	5	3	7	31	NA	Cryo.	No	B	2	2.9	2	4ACL, 4OAU
33.	Bhosale et al.	2007	NA	8	2	6	8	43	14	Cryo.	No	S	3.2	3.8	0	8ACI
34.	Graf et al.	2004	1990–1992	8	8	0	8	32.6	10.5	Cryo.	1No, 7Yes	7S, 1B	9.7	NA	0	8ACL, 1OT, 8ACL+OT
35.	Rueff et al.	2006	NA	8	8	0	8	52	NA	Cryo.	No	B	5.5	NA	0	8ACL
36.	Von Lewinski et al.	2007	1984–1986	6	6	0	6	25	NA	DF	No	S	20	2.6	0	6ACL
37.	Milachowski et al.	1989	NA	22	22	0	22	NA	NA	NA	NA	NA	1, 2	NA	0	22 ACL
38.	Barrett et al. (unpublished data)	1996	NA	15	NA	NA	15	NA	NA	Cryo.	NA	NA	5	NA	NA	NA
39.	Dienst and Kohn											S	3–7			
40.	Kim and Bin	2006	1996–2003	14	NA	NA	14	NA	NA				4.8			

Abbreviations Year P year of publication, *Year S* years of surgery, # number of, *M* number of medial grafts, *L* number of lateral grafts, *Time M-TX* average time in years from meniscectomy to transplantation, *Age* average age of patients at time of transplantation in years
Rad? radiation of graft?, *Preop. Cart.* preoperative cartilage outerbridge grade, *Fix* fixation technique used to fix the allograft, *B* bony fixation, *S* only sutures, *FUT* average time of follow-up in years, # isolated number of transplantation without Concomitant procedures
OT osteotomy, *OAL* osteochondral allograft, *OAU* osteochondral autograft, *ACL* anterior cruciate ligament reconstruction, *PCL* posterior cruciate ligament reconstruction, *MCL* medial collateral ligament reconstruction, *NA* not available, *DF* deep-frozen, *Cryo.* cryopreserved, *Lyo.* lyophilised, *V* viable, *TTT* tuberositas tibiae transfer, *COB* cumulative outerbridge score: calculated by adding the scores for all areas of each knee, *Mi* microfracture, *OPT* osteochondral plug transfer, *ACI* autologous chondrocyte implantation
ODfix osteochondritis dissecans fixation, *CHFC* chondroplasty femoral condyle, *CP* capsular plication, *LR* lateral retinaculum release, *RFA* radiofrequent ablation, *ACPG* articular cartilage past grafting

Table 5.3 Summary of subjective assessment

1.	Cameron et al.	1997	87 % good to excellent rate. (85 % after 3 years) Fulkerson (=modified Lysholm) functional knee score, Tegner score, Reduction in need of anti-inflammatory medication: SI
2.	Carter et al.	1999	IKDC: SI
3.	Goble et al.	1999	Quality of life (regarding pain at rest, during recreational activity and functional stability): SI
4.	Groff et al.	2001	Lysholm score: 91 % fair to excellent ratio
			IKDC: 91 % nearly normal to normal
			All (100 %) were improved, 100 % satisfaction with the condition of their knee as a result of the surgery
			SF-36: 6 of 8 categories higher scoring than age and sex matched population
			KOS at FUT: ADLS: 79.3 SAS: 74.5
			41 % had pain with light sports activities
5.	Wirth et al.	2002	Lysholm, Tegner (at 3y/14y FUT): SI (deep-frozen better than lyophilized, but both deterioration after 14y) (influenced by preoperative cartilage condition and instability)
6.	Noyes et al.	2004	Perception of knee condition: 73 % good to normal. 89 % Improvement of knee function
			76 % Participation in light low-impact sports
			Cincinnati score: SI
7.	Heckmann et al.	2006	94 % improvement of knee condition
			77 % participation in light low-impact sports
8.	Rath et al.	2001	SF-36 for bodily pain, role physical, physical functioning and social functioning: SI
			Mean IKDC functional score: 54
9.	Stollsteimer et al.	2000	Improvement of preoperative pain in 82 %. Tegner score, IKDC score, Lysholm: SI
			Articular cartilage changes preoperatively and preoperatively higher IKDC score had significant effect on overall patient outcome score
10.	Van Arkel et al.	2000	KASS: 84 % successful result
			Modified Lysholm: 84 % fair to excellent
			Tegner: SI
11.	Van Arkel et al.	2002	77 % success
			Lysholm: SI
			91 % improvement of pain

(continued)

Table 5.3 (continued)

12. Verdonk et al.	2005	Relieve in pain and improved function at 10 years in 70 %
13. Verdonk et al.	2006	90 % were satisfied with the operation and would do it again
14. Cole et al.	2006	75 % completely/mostly satisfied with procedure: 68 % medial, 93 % lateral, 81 % isolated, 74 % "combined with other procedure" subgroup
		Lysholm, Tegner, Noyes, IKDC, KOOS pain, symptom, ADL and sports, SF-12 PCS score, VAS pain and overall knee condition: SI
		86 % would have surgery again: 84 % medial subgroup, 93 % lateral subgroup, 86 % isolated and 84 % in combined subgroup
15. Rodeo et al.	1998	88 % of bone plugs + 47 % soft tissue fixated transplantations were rated as GOOD OR MODERATE.
		Lysholm, IKDC, VAS: pain + function: SI
16. Rodeo et al.	2000	58 % clinical successful
17. Del Pizzo et al.	1996	89 % were satisfied with procedure
		95 % Could perform occasional strenuous activities; none continuous
		They all returned to their previous activity level
		Pain was improved in all patients
18. Yoldas et al.	2003	97 % somewhat to greatly improved
		IKDC: 97 % nearly normal to normal
		Lysholm: 68 % good to excellent ratio
		SF-36: in 7 of 8 categories better than age-and sex matched population
19. Ryu et al.		IKDC activity: 68 % nearly normal to normal. VAS, Lysholm II, Tegner score: SI
		Outerbridge grade had significant impact on outcome. 83 % overall satisfaction
20. Hommen et al.		Lysholm, Pain, IKDC, Tegner, SF-12 score: SI. 80 % had improvement
21. L'Insalata	1997	88 % improvement
22. Harner	1993	100 % improvement
23. Felix and Paulos	2002	VAS function: SI
24. Vaquero et al.	2004	VAS pain: SI
		IKDC: 77 % nearly normal to normal

(continued)

Table 5.3 (continued)

25. Sekiya	2006	96 % had improvement of overall function and activity level
		SF-36: PCS and MCS: higher than age- and sex- matched scores from US population
		IKDC: 80 % nearly normal to normal
26. Sekiya	2003	IKDC: 86 % nearly normal to normal (patients with primary ACL reconstruction > revision ACL reconstruction)
		SF-36 PCS and MCS: higher than age- and sex-matched population
		KOS ADLS: 89.7 at FUT, SAS: 81 at FUT
		Lysholm: 88.4 at FUT
		93 % were somewhat to greatly improved
27. Stone	2006	Pain score: SI of 21 %. Self-reported activity scores: SI of 10 %. Self-reported functioning scores: SI of 19 %
		IKDC, WOMAC, Tegner: SI
28. Fukushima	2004	95 % satisfied
		95 % had disappearance of joint line pain. 72 % had disappearance of swelling
29. Rankin	2006	Cincinnati Knee Rating System (pain, patient perception, squatting and run): SI
30. Bhosale et al.	2007	75 % had improvement of function and pain relief at FUT
		Lysholm score: SI
		75 % was satisfied with operation
31. Graf et al.	2004	100 % would recommend procedure to a friend
		88 % continue to actively participate in recreational sports
		IKDC: 50 % nearly normal to normal
32. Rueff et al.	2006	Modified Lysholm, IKDC score, VAS pain: SI
		94 % considered their surgery to be a success and would undergo the procedure again given the same situation
33. Von Lewinski et al.	2007	KOOS at FUT: mean value of 74 points
		Lysholm score: mean value of 74 points at FUT
34. Dienst and Kohn		Joint function and pain reduction: SI

SI significant improvement from preoperatively to follow-up, *FUT* follow-up time

Table 5.4 Objective clinical scoring summary

Nr	Authors	Years	Clinical examination scoring
1.	Groff et al.	2001	91 % no effusion
			mean passive flexion: 129°, NS loss of motion
			side-to side difference in laxity: NS
			0 % had joint line tenderness
			Single leg vertical jump 93 % in comparison to noninvolved limp
			Hop test: 95 % in comparison to noninvolved limp
2.	Noyes and Barber-Westin	2004	3 % had signs of a meniscal tear
			97 % had no tibiofemoral joint-line pain
			89 % had a no effusion
			95 % normal antero-posterior stability
3.	Heckmann et al.	2006	74 % had disappearance of pain at tibiofemoral compartment
4.	Stollsteimer et al.	2000	No patient had loss of motion
5.	Van Arkel et al.	2000	20 % of patients had improvement in stability
6.		2002	20 % of patients had improvement in stability: SI
7.	Verdonk et al.	2005	HSS pain and function: SI
8.		2006	HSS pain score: SI (MMT + HTO group > MMT group)
			HSS walking score: SI
			HSS stair climbing ability score: SI
9.	Cole et al.	2006	IKDC knee examination: 90 % nearly normal to normal at FUT
10.	Rodeo et al.	2001	
11.	Yoldas et al.	2003	81 % no effusion
			100 % no joint line tenderness
			Average flexion at FUT = 129° Average extension at FUT: 2°
			97 % had negative to 1 + Lachmann and pivot shift test at FUT
			vertic jump + hop tests: 85 % compared to contralateral knee
			KT 1000: average side to side difference of 2 mm translation
12.	Hommen et al.	2007	IKDC: 40 % nearly normal to normal

(continued)

Table 5.4 (continued)

Nr	Authors	Years	Clinical examination scoring
13.	Sekiya et al.	2006	IKDC ROM: 31 % nearly normal to normal
			IKDC ligament examination: 94 % nearly normal to normal
			Average loss of flexion compared with non-involved knee: 10°; extension: 4°
			Bony fixation has significant better motion than suture Group
			Single leg hop and vertical jump: 91 % and 85 % of the non-involved leg
14.	Sekiya et al.	2003	IKDC laxity: 92 % nearly normal to normal
			KT-1000: average increase in AP translation of 1.5 mm to contralateral knee
			IKDC ROM: 67 % nearly normal to normal
			Single leg hop and vertical jump: 83 % and 82 % of the non-involved leg
15.	Fukushima et al.	2004	Average ROM + 7° at FUT
16.	Graf et al.	2004	IKDC ROM: 100 % nearly normal to normal
			IKDC ligament examination: 75 % nearly normal to normal
			IKDC compartmental findings: 63 % nearly normal to normal
			IKDC functional test: 75 % nearly normal to normal
			Average loss of motion: 2.3°, average loss of flexion: 4.9°
17.	Von Lewinski et al.	2007	IKDC overall: 40 % nearly normal to normal

FUT follow-up time, *NS* non-significant

5.2.2.2 Radiological Examination

Joint space narrowing indicating cartilage degeneration was observed in a number of patients and tended to increase with a longer duration of follow-up. However, a significant number of patients showed no signs of progression. Based on these limited data, meniscus allograft transplantation is believed to have a chondroprotective effect in 30–40 % of patients. However, the majority of patients are on the 'slippery slope of osteoarthritis' and will further deteriorate over time. It is unknown whether allograft transplantation delays the natural course of osteoarthritis after meniscectomy. Future research is mandatory to determine the chondroprotective power of meniscus allograft transplantation (Table 5.5).

5.2.2.3 MRI Analysis

Routine preoperative MRI may be useful for documentation of articular cartilage defects, subchondral bone status, and any remaining meniscus. Potter et al. [13] demonstrated that MRI provides accurate assessment of meniscal position, horn

Table 5.5 Radiological evaluation

Nr.	Author	Years	FUT (years)	Joint-space narrowing (mean)	Fairbank (average)	IKDC radiological evaluation
1.	Carter et al.	1999	2.9	Progression in 4 %	NA	NA
2.	Garrett et al.	1993	2–3.7	NS	NA	NA
3.	Groff et al.	2001	3.8	NS	NA	NA
4.	Wirth et al.	2002	3 and 14	Increased degenerative changes in all patients	Preoperatively: 0.7. At 3 years: 1.4. At 14 years: 2.5	NA
5.	Noyes et al.	2004	3.3	Progression in 8 %	NA	NA
6.	Rath et al.	2001	4.5	NS	NA	NA
7.	Stollsteimer et al.	2000	3.3	0.88 mm	NA	NA
8.	Verdonk et al.	2006	12.1	Progression in 48 %	Stable in 28 %	NA
9.	Yoldas et al.	2003	2.9	NS increase in joint-space width!	NA	NA
10.	Ryu et al.	2002	2.8	No change in 63 %, 1–3 mm in 25 %, >3 mm in 12.5 %	NA	NA
11.	Hommen et al.	2007	11.7	Progression in 67 %. Mean: 1.15 mm	Progression in 80 %. Mean of 0.8 mm of progression from 0.5 to 1.3	NA
12.	Vaquero et al.	2003	>1	NS	NA	NA
13.	Sekiya et al.	2003	2.8	NS	NA	48 % nearly normal to normal

(continued)

Table 5.5 (continued)

Nr.	Author	Years	FUT (years)	Joint-space narrowing (mean)	Fairbank (average)	IKDC radiological evaluation
14.		2006	3.3	NS	NA	50 % nearly normal to normal
15.	Graf et al.	2004	9.7	Progression in 75 %. Mean of 0,38 mm	NA	12.5 % nearly normal to normal (=same as preoperatively)
16.	Von Lewinski et al.	2007	20	Kellgren-Lawrence score: mean of 2.4	NA	40 % nearly normal to normal
17.	Barrett et al.	1996	5	NS	NA	NA

FUT follow-up time, *NS* not significant
Fairbank changes
Average = zo berekend
Kellgren-Lawrence radiographic grading scale of osteoarthritis of the tibiofemoral joint 0: No radiographic findings of osteoarthritis, 1: Minute osteophytes of doubtful clinical significance, 2: Definite osteophytes with unimpaired joint space, 3: Definite osteophytes with moderate joint space narrowing, 4: Definite osteophytes with severe joint space narrowing and subchondral sclerosis

and capsular attachments, meniscal degeneration and adjacent articular cartilage. It correlates well with arthroscopic evaluation of the transplant and is noninvasive. The development of dynamic and weightbearing MRI shows promise for its use in meniscal transplant analysis (Table 5.6).

In order to overcome the observed discrepancy between clinical outcome and meniscal allograft status and to assess any progression of degenerative articular changes after this type of surgery, objective outcome measures such as MRI have to be included in outcome studies. Only limited literature data are available reporting that meniscal allografting halts or slows down further degeneration [14–17]. In one recent long-term study progression of cartilage degeneration according to MRI and radiological criteria was halted in 35 % of patients, indicating a potential chondroprotective effect [18]. A recent controlled large animal study also confirmed this chondroprotective effect [19]. These data could support the use of prophylactic meniscal transplantation in meniscectomized patients without clinical symptoms, thus potentially limiting secondary cartilage degeneration. Further prospective comparative studies are mandatory to test this hypothesis.

Using MRI, meniscal allograft extrusion has been described independent of the surgical fixation technique. In our experience, using soft-tissue fixation, extrusion is observed in the corpus and anterior horn of the lateral graft, while the posterior horn is most frequently within normal values [18]. This extrusion could reduce the functional surface of the graft and thus potentially also its biomechanical function. Biological reasons for the observed extrusion posttransplantation could include progressive stretch and failure of the circumferential collagen bundle due to insufficient repair potential or increased catabolism. Future research should focus on the biology involved in ongoing metabolic and cellular processes after transplantation.

Lyophilized allografts showed more shrinkage and degeneration, indicated by altered signal intensity, than did other grafts. Therefore, this preservation technique is no longer used. In the long term, all allograft types show some shrinkage. The exact meaning of the observed shrinkage has yet to be determined. Possible hypotheses are tissue loss due to mechanical wear or a biological process of contraction often observed in scar tissue formation and healing.

In general, healing of the allograft to the rim is observed in the vast majority of patients. The meniscus allograft signal is most frequently abnormal with a more greyish appearance. The authors believe that this change in signal reflects biological remodeling of the extracellular matrix of the allograft, rather than true degenerative changes.

5.2.2.4 Second-Look Arthroscopy

Some authors have demonstrated that clinical evaluation only based on symptoms and physical examination does not allow reliable assessment of the status of the meniscus. Arthroscopic evaluation, however, should not be used as a routine postoperative evaluation tool. Most frequently, it is performed upon clinical suspicion of an intra-articular problem. In some cases, arthroscopic evaluation can be performed in association with another procedure around the knee (Table 5.7).

In general, and in accordance with the MRI evaluation, good healing of the allograft to the rim is observed in the vast majority of patients. Tearing and shrinkage can be present. The status of the allograft, however, correlates poorly with the clinical outcome.

5.3 Failures and Survival Analysis

In the literature, no consensus exists on the criteria for failure or success. A number of authors use the clinical outcome, while others propose more objective outcome parameters such as MRI or second-look arthroscopy. In general, using objective parameters, the clinical success rate is higher than estimated. In the majority of studies, a clinical success rate of 70 % and higher has been reported at the final follow-up. Because the success rate has a tendency to decrease over time, it would be preferable to use survivorship analysis rather than failure rate to describe the success of such a procedure. A survivorship is much more powerful to describe the results irrespective of the duration of follow-up. We all are aware that nothing ruins good results more than a long-term follow-up… (Table 5.8).

Based on the available survivorship data, a clinical survivorship of 70 % at 10 years can be anticipated for both medial and lateral allografts. Ligament instability, axial malalignment and cartilage degeneration are considered by most authors to be associated with a higher failure rate and inferior results, although some authors have reported satisfactory results in degenerative knees.

5.4 Conclusion

In conclusion, ample evidence has been presented to support meniscus allograft transplantation in meniscectomized painful knees, with observance of the proper indications. Significant relief of pain and improvement in function have been achieved in a high percentage of patients. These improvements appear to be long-lasting in 70 % of patients. Based on plain radiology and MRI, a subset of patients does not show further cartilage degeneration, indicating a potential chondroprotective effect. The lack of a conservatively treated control group is considered a fundamental flaw in the reported studies, making it difficult to establish the true chondroprotective effect of this type of treatment.

Based on the presented results, meniscus allograft transplantation should no longer be considered experimental surgery for the meniscectomized painful knee.

Table 5.6 MRI Analysis

Nr.	Author	Years	FUT (years)	MRI
1.	Wirth et al.	2002	14	*Deep-frozen allografts*
				– showed good preservation, no reduction in size, homogenous signal
				– showed chondromalacia grade 2
				Lyophilized allografts
				– were reduced in size, had altered signal intensity (=degeneration)
				– showed chondromalacia grade 2 in 16 %, grade 3 in 67 % and grade 4 in 16 %
2.	Noyes et al.	2004	3.3	In the coronal plane:
				– mean displacement: 2.2 mm
				– 59 % of the allografts had no displacement
				Intrameniscal signal intensity: 4 % normal, 46 % grade 1, 39 % grade 2, 11 % grade 3
3.	Stollsteimer et al.	2000	2	42 % had an abnormal mri signal, but no tear
				Average size of meniscus was 62 % of the normal meniscus (graft shrinkage)
				9 % had 1 mm extrusion
4.	Van Arkel et al.	2000	2.7	63 % completely healed to the capsule, 26 % partially detached, 11 % total detached
				21 % showed severe shrinkage, 21 % moderate shrinkage
				0 % had a normal position: 11 % bucket-handle-like configuration, 32 % extrusion, 58 % subextrusion

(continued)

Table 5.6 (continued)

Nr.	Author	Years	FUT (years)	MRI
5.	Verdonk et al.	2006	12	No progression of cartilage degeneration in 35 %
				No changes in signal intensity of the allograft: in 82 %
				No change in graft position in 35 %
				Tear observed in 12 %
6.		2004	1	The lateral transplanted meniscus is more extruded in comparison to the normal lateral meniscus.; The anterior horn (mean 5.8 mm) seems to be more extruded than the posterior horn (mean 2.7 mm)
7.	Hommen et al.	2007	11.7	71 % had grade 3 signal intensities
				57 % had moderately truncated mid-zones; 29 % had moderately diminutive anterior horns, 14 % had a severely truncated mid zone
				100 % moderate graft shrinkage
				Cartilage classification: 14 % normal, 29 % mild, 43 % moderate and 14 % severe
8.	Vaquero et al.	2003	>1	5 % changes in signal intensity
9.	Potter et al.	1996	1	– 63 % showed increased signal intensity in the posterior horn tibial attachment (=degenerative changes)
				– moderate (4) or severe (11) chondral degeneration in 63 %
				– 46 % showed peripheral displacement
				– Fragmentation (21 %) and frank extrusion (12.5 %) were associated with full-thickness chondral loss
10.	Rankin et al.	2006	2	– the mean height and width of the anterior and posterior horns were similar to native menisci
				– MRI under weight-bearing conditions
				– The anterior horn of the native meniscus moved a mean of 5 mm compared to allograft
				– Signal intensity: 25 % grade 1, 50 % grade 2, 25 % grade 3

(continued)

Table 5.6 (continued)

Nr.	Author	Years	FUT (years)	MRI
11.	Bhosale et al.	2007	1	Good integration in all, no rejection
				Mild extrusion in 20 %
				63 % wedge shaped, 25 % flat, 12 % expansion
				50 % had blurred surface
				100 % had increased signal intensity
12.	Von Lewinski et al.	2007	20	Transplants showed shrinkage, degenerative changes
				17 % subluxation
				Osteophytes

Stoller et al. classification Grade 1 represented a nonarticular focal or globular intrasubstance focus of increased signal, *grade 2* represented linear focus of intrasubstance increased signal that extended from the capsular periphery of the meniscus but did not involve an articular meniscal surface, and *grade 3* represented an area of increased signal intensity that communicated or extended to at least 1 articular surface

Extrusion of the allograft the portion of the allograft that was displaced completely over the peripheral border of the tibial plateau

Subextrusion portion of the allograft that was displaced partially over the peripheral border of the tibial plateau

Table 5.7 Evaluation by second-look arthroscopy

Nr.	Author	Years	FUT (years)	
1.	Cameron et al.	1997	2.5	77 % complete healing, 23 % failed healing, 0 % shrinkage, 60 % postop. Posterior horn tear
2.	Carter et al.	1999	2.8	18 % failed healing, 14 % shrinkage
				9 % arthritis progression
3.	Garrett et al.	1993	2	71 % complete healing
4.	Goble et al.	1999	2	72 % intact
5.	Wirth et al.	2002	3.8	– deepfrozen: 40 % shrinkage, 100 % complete healing.
				– lyophilized: 14 % incomplete healing/detachment and 93 % showed shrinkage
				– 91 % complete healing
6.	Noyes et al.	1998	1.3	8 % complete healing, 31 % partial healing, 57 % failed healing
				29 % showed degeneration/tears
7.		2004	3.3	56 % failed healing/degeneration/tears
				Articular cartilage: 85 % abnormal
8.	Rath et al.	2001	2.6	100 % complete healing
				80 % had degeneration/tears
				Arthroscopy was only performed in case of symptoms
9.	Stollsteimer et al.	2000	3.3	4 % loosening
10.	Van Arkel et al.	2000	2.7	79 % complete healing, 16 % partial healing, 5 % failed healing
				58 % subextrusion, 11 %extrusion, 11 % bucket-handle
				21 % shrinkage
				Articular cartilage: 50 % grade 3, 38 % grade 3–4, 12, 5 % grade 4 outerbridge
11.	Verdonk et al.	2005	7.2	Menisci with poor function or persist pain had severe allograft degeneration or allograft detachment
12.	Shelton and Dukes	1994	NA	100 % complete healing
13.	Veltri et al.	1994	0.5	71 % complete healing, 29 % partial healing
				14 % showed degeneration

(continued)

Table 5.7 (continued)

Nr.	Author	Years	FUT (years)	
14.	Del Pizzo et al.	1996	3.2	100 % showed complete healing
				6 % showed tear
15.	Yoldas et al.	2003	0.5–1	100 % complete healing
				33 % radial tear <1 cm
16.	Ryu et al.	2002	2.75	50 % complete healing
				20 % degeneration/tear
17.	Cryolife	1997	7	91 % fully intact in bone block cases
18.	Vaquero et al.	2003	>1	20 % shrinkage
				20 % loosening
19.	Potter et al.	1996	1	58 % subextrusion, 16 % extrusion
				26 % degeneration (fragmentation)
				Only patients with frank displacement on MRI were confirmed at arthroscopic evaluation
				52 % focal synovitis at the peripheral capsular attachment
				All areas that were seen as moderate-to-fullthickness chondral degeneration, were confirmed on arthroscopy as OB grade 3–4 change
20.	Stone et al.	2006	5.8	21 % torn menisci
21.	Bhosale et al.	2007	1	100 % complete healing
				12,5 % meniscus thinning
				25 % mild synovitis
22.	Graf et al.	2004	4	100 % complete healing
				33 % had a tear
				loose body removal in one case
				100 % well-vascularized
				No progression of degenerative changes

Table 5.8 Failure criteria and failure rate

Nr.	Author	Years	Rehabilitation program
1.	Cameron et al.	1997	Week 1–3: immobilization
			Week 3–6: progressive ROM (first 6 weeks nwb)
			From week 6: quadriceps and hamstrings exercises
2.	Groff et al.	2001	First week: pwb (crutches) with immobilization in extension-brace; cpm machine for 3 weeks; full extension at one week
			Second week: passive and active ROM of 0–90°; brace unlocked; weight-bearing as tolerated
			Week 4–6: 90°, crutches discontinued
			From week 6: closed chain exercises
			From week 8: low-impact sports
			Rehabilitation of 2–3 months
			Return to strenuous work at 3–4 months, to running at 4–5 months
			Return to strenuous sports not encouraged
3.	Wirth et al.	2002	Immediately after surgery: CPM and physical therapy
			Week 1–12: rehabilitation program
			Week 13: fwb
4.	Noyes et al.	2004	Immediately postoperative: long leg brace for 8 weeks; ROM 0–90° exercises from the first day; flexibility and quadriceps exercises
			Flexion increased every week by 10° to allow 135° after week 4
			Week 1–2: only toe-touch wb, increased to 50 % wb after week 4
			Week 6: fwb; balance, proprioception and closed chain exercises
			Week 8: stationary cycling with low resistance
			Week 9–12: swimming and walking programs
			After 12 months: light recreational sports
			Advised to never return to high-impact strenuous athletics again
			If PCL reconstruction: restricted in flexion and wb for 8 weeks
			If ACL reconstruction: other protocol
			Bledsoe Thruster brace when abnormal articular cartilage
5.	Rath et al.	2001	From day 1: quadriceps and hamstrings exercises, limited ROM 0–90°
			Week 1–4: nwb
			Week 4–6: pwb
			6–9 months: full activity
			Never aggressive cutting sports or distance running again

(continued)

Table 5.8 (continued)

Nr.	Author	Years	Rehabilitation program
6.	Stollsteimer et al.	2000	Immediately postoperatively: full ROM exercises
			Week 1–6: no fwb
			jogging at 3 months, sports at 6 months
7.	Verdonk et al.	2005	Week 1–3: nwb with ROM flexion to max 60°
			Week 3–6: ROM 0–90° + pwb
			From week 6: walk with 1 crutch
8.		2006	Week 1–3: nwb with ROM flexion to max 60°
			Week 3–6: ROM 0–90° + pwb
			From week 6: walk with 1 crutch
9.	Shelton and Dukes	1994	Immediately postoperative: full ROM, nwb till week 6
			From day 1: quadriceps and hamstrings exercises
			Week 6: fwb
			6 months: return to sports if knee is fully rehabilitated
10.	Veltri et al.	1994	Week 1–6: pwb + ROM exercises in hinged brace
			After week 6 fwb as tolerated
11.	Cole et al.	2006	Immediately postoperative: wb as tolerated with crutches + hinged brace + immediate active and passive ROM without limitation
			Week 1–6: flexion wb < 90° restricted
			After week 6: no brace + ROM as tolerated
			After 12 weeks: jogging allowed with progression to running and sport-specific-type drills
12.	Yoldas et al.	2003	Immediately postoperative: quadriceps sets and straight leg raises
			Day 1: start passive ROM with CPM, for 1 month
			Week 1: full extension, pwb, brace locked in extension
			From week 2: wb as tolerated
			Week 4–6: 90° flexion, fwb, closed chain exercises
			Rehabilitation of 2–3 months
13.	Ryu et al.	2002	Immobilization in full extension with progressive wb over 4–5 weeks
			Week 1–4: ROM 0–90°
			From week 5: gradual increase in flexion of 10–15° each week
			If concomitant ACL reconstruction: ACL protocol was subordinated to meniscal allografts requirements

(continued)

Table 5.8 (continued)

Nr.	Author	Years	Rehabilitation program
14.	Hommen et al.	2007	Immediately postoperative: quadriceps sets en straight leg raising
			24 h after surgery CPM till 1 month
15.	Felix and Paulos	2002	Postoperatively braced in extension. Plantar touch wb
			Week 3: 60° flexion
			Week 4: progressive wb increased by 25 % every week
			Week 6: full flexion
			Week 7–8: fwb
			6–9 months: full activities and sports
16.	Sekiya et al.	2003	Immediately postoperative: exercises, pwb with crutches, brace locked in full extension
			Day 1: cpm
			Week 1: full extension
			Week 2: wb as tolerated, sedentary work
			Week 4–6: 90° flexion, stop crutches
			From week 6: close chain exercises
			strenuous work and running after 5–6 months—sports after 6–9 months
17.		2006	Immediately postoperative: exercises, pwb with crutches, brace locked in full extension
			Day 1: cpm
			Week 1: full extension
			Week 2: wb as tolerated, sedentary work
			Week 4–6: 90° flexion, stop crutches
			From week 6: close chain exercises
			strenuous work and running after 5–6 months—sports after 6–9 months
18.	Stone et al.	2006	Week 1–4: MAXIMAL PROTECTIVE PHASE = pwb (week 1 and 2: 10 and 20 % toe touch), extension-locked hinged brace, passive and active ROM, daily icing and elevation, straight leg exercises, manually resisted hip, foot and ankle exercises, pool workouts, soft-tissue treatments, a trunk stabilization program, nwb aerobic exercises
			Week 4–12: MODERATE PROTECTIVE PHASE = stretching, manual treatments to restore ROM, the introduction of functional
			exercises (i.e., partial squats, calf raises, and Proprioception exercises), road cycling as tolerated, slow walking on a low-impact treadmill, and lateral training. Exercises increasingly focus on single-leg exercises, strength training, and sport-specific training for a gradual return to activities
			No resisted leg extension machines, no high-impact, cutting, or twisting activities for at least 4 months postoperatively

(continued)

Table 5.8 (continued)

Nr.	Author	Years	Rehabilitation program
19.	Fukushima et al.	2004	24-48 h postoperative: start ROM exercises
			Week 1–4: nwb
			Week 5: pwb 50 %
			Week 6: fwb + Flexion > 90° allowed
			Week 8–10: Closed chain exercises
			Never strenuous/contact/rotational sports in the future
20.	Rankin et al.	2006	Postoperatively: long leg brace for 6 weeks, ROM 0–90°, toe-touch wb first 2 weeks, flexibility and quadriceps strengthening exercises
			Week 3–4: flexion to 120°, 50 % wb
			Week 5–6: ROM 0°–135° at 4 weeks
			Week 6: fwb + balance, Proprioception, closed kinetic chain exercises
			Week 7–8: stationary cycling
			Week 9–12: start swimming and walking
			12 Months: light recreational sports
			Never high-impact activities/strenuous athletics again
21.	Bhosale et al.	2007	The Oscell Rehabilitation for ACI procedure and limit of knee flexion to 45° for 3 weeks
			Week 12: fwb
22.	Graf et al.	2004	Week 1–2: nwb, light resistive isometric exercises, medial unloading brace 10–90° (if + ACL reconstruction: derotational brace), stationary biking when 90° was obtained
			Week 2–4: pwb
			Week 5: fwb
			Week 6: resistance exercises
			3 months: advancement in rehabilitation exercises and strengthening programs
			6 months: stop bracing, start straight line jogging (without cutting and pivoting)
			8 months: start agility exercises
			1 year: sporting activities (never high-impact, running, jumping, twisting or turning sports again)
23.	Rueff et al.	2006	Week 1–6: ROM limited to 0–90°
			Early wb

(continued)

Table 5.8 (continued)

Nr.	Author	Years	Rehabilitation program
24.	Von Lewinski et al.	2007	Postoperatively: strengthening exercises for quadriceps muscle, brace with limited ROM for 12 weeks
			Week 1–6: ROM 30–60°
			Week 6–12: ROM 20–90°
			Week 1–12: pwb 10 kg
25.	Dienst and Kohn		Postoperatively: ROM 0–90° active + passive exercises, pwb with brace locked in extension for 6 weeks
			3 months: now full squat allowed
			1 year: sport activities allowed

ROM range of motion
nwb non-weight bearing
cpm continuous passive motion
pwb partial weight-bearing
fwb full weight bearing
wb weight bearing
The Oscell rehabilitation for ACI procedure

References

1. Cameron JC, Saha S (1997) Meniscal allograft transplantation for unicompartmental arthritis of the knee. Clin Orthop 337:164–171
2. Noyes FR, Barber-Westin SD (1995) Irradiated meniscus allografts in the human knee: a two to five year follow-up study. Orthop Trans 19:417
3. Verdonk PCM, Demurie A, Almqvist KF, Veys EM, Verbruggen, Verdonk R (2005) Transplantation of viable meniscal allograft: survivorship analysis and clinical outcome of one hundred cases. J Bone Joint Surg Am 87:715–724
4. Ryu RK, Dunbar VWH, Morse GG (2002) Meniscal allograft replacement: a 1-year to 6-year experience. Arthroscopy 18:989–994
5. Stone KR, Walgenbach AW, Turek TJ, Freyer A, Hill MD (2006) Meniscus allograft survival in patients with moderate to severe unicompartmental arthritis: a 2- to 7-year follow-up. Arthroscopy 22(5):469–478
6. Bhosale AM, Myint P, Roberts S, Menage J, Harrison P, Ashton B, Smith T, McCall I, Richardson JB (2007) Combined autologous chondrocyte implantation and allogenic meniscus transplantation: a biological knee replacement. Knee 14(5):361–368
7. Walker PS, Erkman MJ (1975) The role of the menisci in force transmission across the knee. Clin Orthop 109:184–192
8. Johnson DL, Bealle D (1999) Meniscal allograft transplantation. Clin Sports Med 18:93–108
9. Cole BJ, Carter TR, Rodeo SA (2003) Allograft meniscal transplantation: background, techniques, and results. Instr Course Lect 52:383–396
10. Rodeo SA (2001) Meniscal allografts—where do we stand? Am J Sports Med 29:246–261
11. Cole BJ, Cohen B (2000) Chondral injuries of the knee. A contemporary view of cartilage restoration. Orthop Spec Ed 6:71–76
12. Rijk PC (2004) Meniscal allograft transplantation—part i: background, results, graft selection and preservation, and surgical considerations. Arthroscopy 20:728–743

13. Potter HG, Rodeo SA, Wickiewicz TL et al (1996) MR imaging of meniscal allografts: correlation with clinical and arthroscopic outcomes. Radiology 198:509–514
14. Zukor DJ, Cameron JC, Brooks PJ et al (1990) The fate of human meniscal allografts. In: Ewing JW (ed) Articular cartilage and knee joint function. Raven, New York, pp 147–152
15. Garrett JC (1993) Meniscal transplantation: a review of 43 cases with 2- to 7- year follow-up. Sports Med Arthrosc Rev 1:164–167
16. Kuhn JE, Wojtys EM (1996) Allograft meniscal transplantation. Clin Sports Med 15:537–556
17. Stollsteimer GT, Shelton WR, Dukes A, Bomboy AL (2000) Meniscal allograft transplantation: a 1-to-5 year follow-up of 22 patients. Arthroscopy 16:343–347
18. Verdonk PCM, Demurie A, Almqvist KF, Veys EM, Verbruggen G, Verdonk R (2006) Transplantation of viable meniscal allograft. J Bone Joint Surg Am 88(1 Suppl 1):109–118
19. Aagaard H, Jorgensen U, Bojsen-Moller F (2003) Immediate versus delayed meniscal allograft transplantation in sheep. Clin Orthop 406:218–227

Part II
Meniscal Substitutes

Collagen Meniscal Implant (CMI)

6

Joan Carles Monllau

6.1 Basic Science

Joan Carles Monllau[1]
Marc Tey[2]
Erquicia[3]

6.1.1 Introduction

The meniscus performs critical physiological as well as biomechanical functions within the knee. It distributes loads across adjacent articular cartilage thereby protecting the hyaline cartilage from wear. Meniscal tears are one of the most common injuries of this joint leading to the surgical excision of the injured tissue in most of the cases. However, it is well known since the pioneering works of King [1] and Fairbank [2] that the loss of meniscal tissue frequently leads to osteoarthritis and irreversible joint damage. The advent of arthroscopic partial

J. C. Monllau (✉)
Department of Orthopaedic Surgery, Hospital de la Sta Creu i Sant Pau, ICATME—Institut Universitari Dexeus, Universitat Autònoma de Barcelona, Sant Antoni Maria Claret, 167, 08025, Barcelona, Spain
e-mail: Jmonllau@santpau.cat

[1] Department of Orthopaedic Surgery, Hospital de la Sta Creu i Sant Pau, ICATME—Institut Universitari Dexeus, Universitat Autònoma de Barcelona, Sant Antoni Maria Claret, 167, 08025 Barcelona, Spain. e-mail: jmonllau@santpaqu.cat

[2] ICATME. Institut Universitari Dexeus, Universitat Autònoma de Barcelona, Sabino Arana 5-19, 08028 Barcelona, Spain. e-mail: Mtey.icatme@idexeus.es

[3] ICATME. Institut Universitari Dexeus, Universitat Autònoma de Barcelona, Sabino Arana 5-19, 08028 Barcelona, Spain. e-mail: juanerquicia@yahoo.com

R. Verdonk et al. (eds.), *Meniscal Transplantation*,
DOI: 10.1007/978-3-642-38106-5_6, © ISAKOS 2013

meniscectomy contributed to improve these results. Nevertheless, the long-term follow-up still shows that a substantial number of patients suffered the effect of a lost meniscus [3, 4].

In an effort to keep the knee joint functional and pain free, a renewed interest in meniscal preservation techniques appeared in the last three decades. Due to the poor ability of prosthetic replacement to reproduce the meniscus behavior and the limited availability of allografts, tissue engineering techniques were developed for the same purpose. The Collagen Meniscus Implant (CMI. ReGen Biologics, Hackensack, New Jersey, USA) is a collagen based meniscus implant consisting in a resorbable scaffold designed to support ingrowths of new tissue to eventually regenerate the lost meniscus. It is a biologically resorbable implant with a spongy texture consisting of a highly purified type I collagen. The CMI was developed from bovine collagen in the early 90s in order to promote regeneration in segmental defects of meniscal tissue [5]. Stone et al. [6, 7], firstly demonstrated the ability of the implant to regenerate meniscal tissue in both dogs and humans.

To date, experimental and clinical experiences with the medial CMI have shown promising results [7–11] and a lateral implant has been developed and recently tested in several European centres.

The purpose of this chapter is to describe the CMI background and surgical technique along with some tricks and limitations gleaned from the author's experience of 15 years with its use that might help the reader to achieve the most successful outcome. The ten-year results of a medial CMI series are also presented.

6.1.2 Background

Collagen matrices, acting as templates for the growth of fibrous tissue, were developed in the early eighty's with different purposes [12–14]. Following the same investigational line, a resorbable collagen meniscus implant (CMI) was developed to support the regeneration of meniscal tissue. Experimental studies in a canine model showed that the scaffold was able to support substantial meniscal regeneration while slowly reabsorbed. In these studies, the regenerated neo-meniscus had a histological and biochemical appearance that was similar to that of original canine meniscal fibrocartilage [5, 6]. Genovese et al. [15] have recently characterized the ultrastructure of the implant at a minimum of 6 moths after implantation. These biopsy findings demonstrate that host cells (likely derived from the adjacent synovium) migrate into the collagen meniscus scaffold, differentiate into fibroblast-like cells, and synthesize appropriate extracellular matrix.

6.1.3 The Implant

The CMI was conceived to conduct meniscal regeneration in the early 80s. It has physical size and shape approximating the original human meniscus. The implants are made of type I collagen fibres derived from bovine Achilles tendon. After the tendon tissue is trimmed and minced, the type I collagen fibres are purified by using various chemical treatments to remove non-collagenous proteins and lipids. Next, the purified collagen fibres are swelled in hyaluronic acid and chondroitin sulphate and then homogenized. The swollen collagen fibres plus the glycosaminoglycans are co-precipitated by the addition of ammonium hydroxide. The precipitated fibres are dehydrated, manually oriented in a mould, lyophilized, and chemically cross-linked. Finally, terminal sterilization is performed by γ irradiation [5].

6.1.4 Patient Selection Criteria

The CMI is not a prosthetic device. It is intended to provide a resorbable scaffold that will be replaced by the patient's own tissue over time. Unlike meniscus allografts that are used to replace the entire meniscus, the CMI is designed to solely replace the damaged or missing portion of the meniscus. The ideal patient must have an intact meniscal rim and anterior and posterior horns for a good attachment and stability of the scaffold. Otherwise, would not accomplish the hoop stress law and the final construct will be extruded from the tibial plateau, resulting in a non-effective procedure. In addition, the surgically prepared site for the CMI must extend at least into the red-white zone of the meniscus to provide sufficient vascular supply.

Patients were excluded if they had had a previous treatment with collagen or if they had an allergy to collagen, inflammatory arthritis or degenerative joint disease and evidence of osteonecrosis in the targeted area. It is also contraindicated in patients allergic to bovine or other animal derived products, with an overly sensitized immune system, systemic or local infection.

6.2 Surgical Technique and Results

Joan Carles Monllau[4]
Xavier Pelfort[5]

6.2.1 Surgical Technique Tips and Tricks

The operative technique for implantation included an arthroscopic evaluation of the knee joint by the standard antero-lateral and antero-medial approaches. After identifying the meniscal tear, the removal of only the irreparably damaged tissue is

[4] Department of Orthopaedic Surgery, Hospital de la Sta Creu i Sant Pau, ICATME- Institut Universitari Dexeus, Universitat Autònoma de Barcelona, Sant Antoni Maria Claret, 167, 08025 Barcelona, Spain. e-mail: jmonllau@santpaqu.cat

[5] Department of Orthopaedic Surgery, Parc de Salut Mar, Universitat Autònoma de Barcelona, Paseig Maritim 25, 08003 Barcelona, Spain. e-mail: jpelfort@parcdesalutmar.cat

performed, leaving a rim and the anterior and posterior limits square (Fig 6.1). A bleeding bed was created at the periphery by debridement into the vascular zone. If a healthy meniscal rim is achieved in the red-white zone, in order to guarantee a good vascular supply the surgeon must do a meniscal trephination (Fig 6.2). This can be performed either by passing an 18 gauge spinal needle from outside-in multiple times or conversely using a micro-fracture awl from inside-out. The created channels can also contribute for cellular in-growth. If a valgus force is applied while needling it may facilitate the partial release of the medial collateral ligament thus diminishing scuffing the articular cartilage and facilitating the whole procedure in case of medial tight knee.

The missing or removed area of the meniscus is then measured with a calibrated Teflon rod to estimate the size of the implant that was needed (Fig 6.3). The implant is prepared according to the determined defect size although over-sizing it by 3–5 mm, to get a good press fit between implant and meniscus remnant in the final construct. The implant is then inserted through the previously enlarged (about 2 cm) antero-medial or antero-lateral portal using a vascular clamp (Fig 6.4). To facilitate this manoeuvre, the surgeon stops the inflow (dry insertion) thus avoiding the flip-out of the scaffold into the joint. Then a secure attachment of the implant to the remaining host meniscus must be obtained. To this end, either an inside–out or an all-inside technique can be used. If the inside-out method is to be used, a complete set of zone specific cannulae as well as an additional posterior approach or several small stab wounds to retrieve the suturing needles are necessary (Fig 6.5). As for any meniscal repair, 2.0 non-absorbable sutures are recommended. Vertical mattress sutures all along the meniscus rim and horizontal sutures at the anterior and posterior ends of the implant were preferred (Fig 6.6) The stitches were placed every 5 mm apart and tied directly over the posterior part of the medial or lateral aspect of the capsule, depending on the meniscus to be

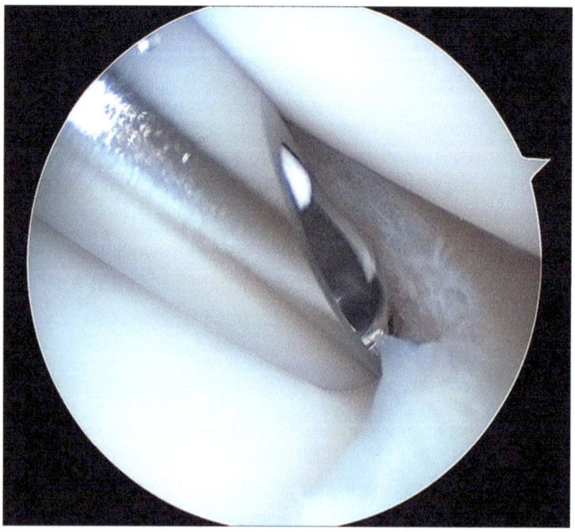

Fig. 6.1 Meticulous preparation of the implant bed with removal of damaged tissue to guarantee a stable rim in which the implant can be properly fixed

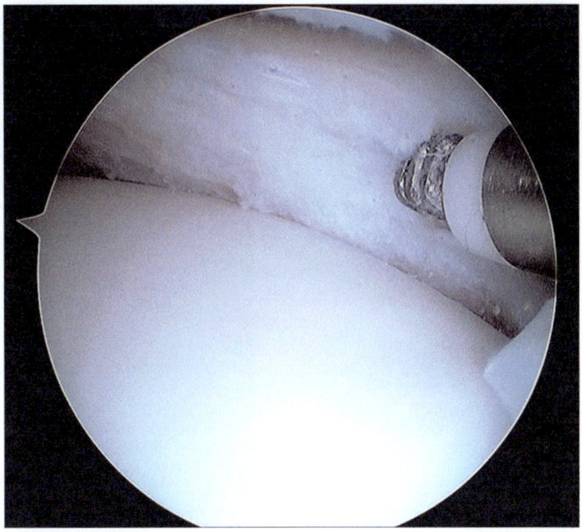

Fig. 6.2 High frequency trephination of the synovial and meniscal bed in order to guarantee a vascular supply. Note the anterior limit of the meniscal defect trimmed square

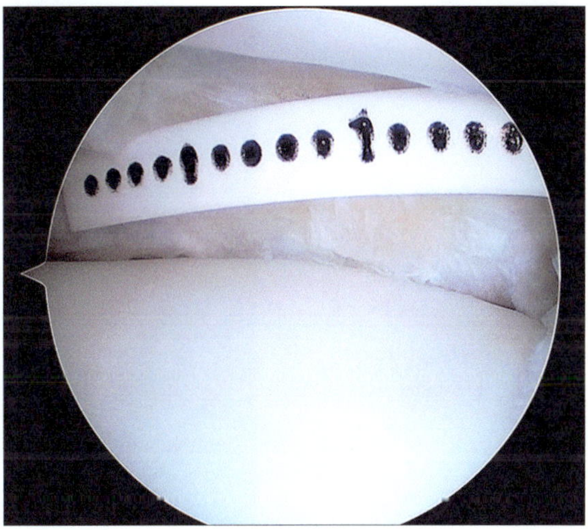

Fig. 6.3 A calibrated Teflon rod is used to measure the dimension of the defect and thus the size of the implant to be used

repaired [16]. However, if the surgeon uses an all-inside suture system (i.e. Fastfix, S&N, Andover, USA) more room between the stitches, about 1 cm, seems to be also adequate.

6.2.2 Especial Situations

Knee instability or axial malalignment in the lower extremity are common associated problems. ACL reconstruction can be performed concurrently with the CMI implantation. In that case, the tunnels for the ACL reconstruction are drilled first

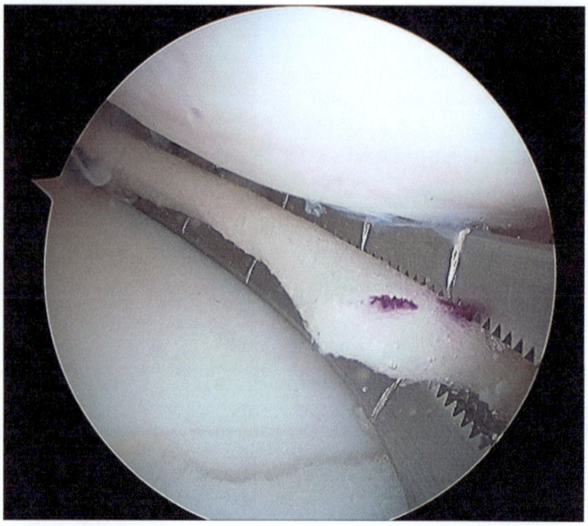
Fig. 6.4 Dry insertion of the CMI using a *vascular clamp*

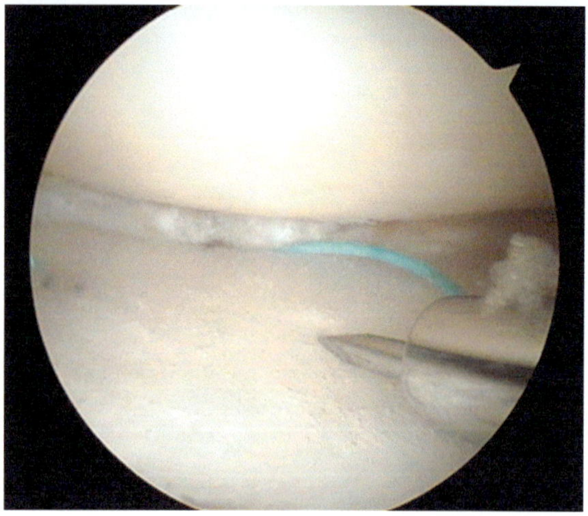
Fig. 6.5 Inside-out suture using zone specific cannulae

and the graft is passed and secured at the femoral site. Then the surgeon proceeds with the meniscal implant avoiding any over tension in the involved compartment. Once the implant has been correctly secured the knee is drawn to 20° of flexion and the ACL graft fixed at the tibial site.

If the procedures are to be staged, the CMI implantation typically should be performed first. The ACL reconstruction should be completed within 12 weeks after CMI implantation since knee instability is detrimental to the implant as noted.

If there is axial malalignment of the lower extremity, it should be corrected before or at least concurrently with the placement of the implant. Malalignment may excessively overload the involved compartment, possibly resulting in damage

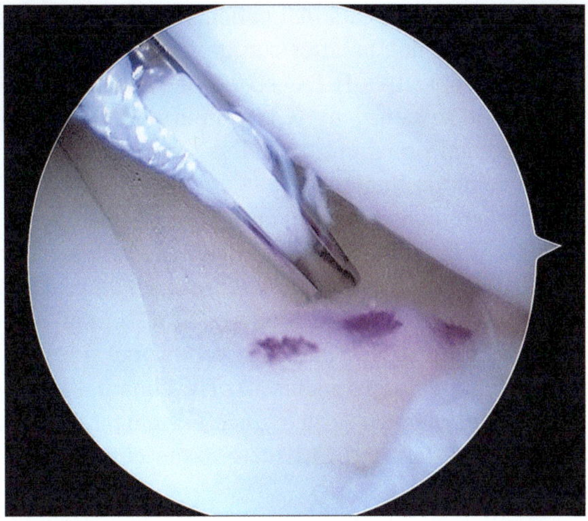

Fig. 6.6 The all-inside suturing system used at the anterior end of the implant

to the implant during the early regenerative process. No controlled studies have been conducted to confirm this possibility. Whether or not there is a coexisting OA with the malalignment, consideration should be given to correcting those abnormalities prior to or at least concurrent with the CMI implantation.

If the osteotomy and the implant procedures are done concurrently, consideration must be given to the CMI-specific rehabilitation program.

6.2.3 Rehabilitation

The rehabilitation protocol was defined as follows: patients had to wear a knee brace locked at full extension and were non-weight bearing for the initial 2 weeks while using crutches to walk. The brace could be removed to perform passive range of motion (ROM) exercises. After 4 week, the brace was discontinued for unlimited active and passive ROM exercises and patients increased weight bearing up to full weight bearing by the 6th week. After 8 weeks, patients discontinued the use of crutches. Strengthening exercises progressed from right after surgery until patients returned to full unrestricted activity. Return to sports was not recommended earlier than 6 months after CMI implantation.

6.2.4 Results

Several clinical non-randomized follow-ups have studied the collagen based implant and observed a re-growth of meniscal-like tissue and improvement of knee function overtime in a significant number of cases. Zaffagnini et al. prospectively evaluated the results of a short series of 8 patients after CMI implantation at a follow up of 6–8 years. All patients were able to return to daily activities without limitations 3 months after surgery. Both the subjective Cinncinatti Knee Rating Scale and objective IKDC scores showed improvement in all but one case. The patient had sustained an ACL re-injury. MRI showed an altered signal in five cases and a normal signal in two. In this series, a reduction in the implants expected size was a common finding.

Bulgheroni et al. have also investigated the medial CMI in a series of 34 patients with radiological and magnetic resonance imaging. Lysholm and Tegner activity scores at 2–5 years after surgery improved significantly compared to the preoperative scores. The MRI signal also improved over time after implantation. There was a progressive decrease in signal intensity but it was not comparable to the signal of a normal meniscus. The chondral surfaces of the medial compartment had not degenerated further since placement of the CMI. If compared to a normal medial meniscus, the CMI-new tissue complex had a slight reduction in size in most cases.

Monllau et al. followed-up 25 patients who underwent arthroscopic implantation of the collagen meniscus device. Indications were persistent compartmental joint line pain due to a previous medial meniscus resection (5 cases) or a large irreparable meniscus tear found at arthroscopy (20 cases). It was possible to evaluate 22 patients at a minimum of 10 years after the procedure. The improvement of clinical functional scales and pain was considered highly significant at 1 year follow-up and the results have remained unchanged over time. Radiographic evaluation showed either minimal or no narrowing of the joint line at the most recent follow-up. According to the Genovese criteria [15], magnetic resonance imaging showed meniscus type 2 in two-thirds of the cases. Again, all cases showed a new meniscus of less volume than expected. The failure rate in the patient population was 8 % (2 of 25). There were no complications related to the device.

Recently, Zaffagnini et al. [17] analyzed a series of 33 patients with meniscal injuries at 5–10 years after surgery. Some of the patients were non-randomly treated with a medial CMI while the rest (matched controls) were treated with partial meniscectomy. The CMI group showed a significantly lower VAS for pain, and a higher objective IKDC, Tegner index and SF-36 scores when compared with the partial meniscectomy group. Radiographic evaluation also showed significantly less medial joint space narrowing in the CMI group. The MRI evaluation of the CMI patients revealed 11 cases of myxoid degeneration signal. Therefore, in this series the CMI treatment seems to be superior to meniscectomy in terms of pain, activity level, and radiological outcomes at a minimum 10-year follow-up when compared with partial meniscectomy alone.

This information was further refined by the large study conducted by Rodkey et al. [18]. These authors published a prospective multicenter randomized controlled trial comparing medial CMI with partial medial meniscectomy at an average of 5 years follow-up. Three hundred and eleven patients with meniscal problems were divided into two study arms. One group was considered acute, meaning patients without previous surgery to the involved meniscus. The second group was chronic, those patients having had one or more prior meniscectomies. They were randomly assigned either to receive a collagen meniscus implant or to have a partial meniscectomy. Patients receiving a CMI agreed to have a second look arthroscopy at one-year after implantation to assess the amount and quality of the new tissue growth. According to the Tegner score, chronic patients receiving an implant regained significantly more of their lost activity than did controls and they had significantly fewer reoperations in the involved knee. However, no differences were detected between the two treatments in acute patients. On the other hand second-look arthroscopies performed 1 year after implantation demonstrated that the CMI supports the formation of a new biomechanically competent meniscus-like tissue.

6.3 Summary

According to the available literature, meniscal substitution with the CMI provides significant pain relief and functional improvement after a minimum of 10 years' follow-up. The implant generally diminished in size, but the procedure proved to be safe and had a low rate of implant failure on a long-term basis. No development or progression of degenerative knee joint disease was observed in most cases. The most benefit seems to appear in symptomatic patients with a previous meniscectomy, particularly when the implantation is compared with a new iterative meniscectomy.

Although the CMI is safe for the joint and had no apparent negative effects, the efficacy of this device in reducing the risk of degenerative disease remains to be proven.

References

1. King D (1936) The function of semilunar cartilages. J Bone Joint Surg 18A:1069
2. Fairbank TD (1948) Knee joint changes after meniscectomy. J Bone Joint Surg 30-B:664–670
3. Burks RT, Metcalf MH, Metcalf RW (1997) Fifteen-year follow-up of arthroscopic partial meniscectomy. Arthroscopy 13(6):673–679
4. Higuchi H, Kimura M, Shirakura K, Terauchi M, Takagishi K (2000) Factors affecting long-term results after arthroscopic partial meniscectomy. Clin Orthop Relat Res 377:161–168
5. Stone KR, Rodkey WG, Webber RJ et al (1990) Future directions: collagen-based prostheses for meniscal regeneration. Clin Orthop 252:129–135
6. Stone KR, Rodkey WG, Webber RJ et al (1992) Meniscal regeneration with copolymeric collagen scaffolds. In vitro and in vivo studies evaluated clinically, histologically, and biochemically. Am J Sports Med 20:104–111
7. Stone KR, Steadman JR, Rodkey WG, Li S-T (1997) Regeneration of meniscal cartilage with use of a collagen scaffold. Analysis of preliminary data. J Bone Joint Surg Am 79:1770–1777
8. Steadman JR, Rodkey WG (2005) Tissue-engineered collagen meniscus implants: 5- to 6-year feasibility study results. Arthroscopy 21(5):515–525

9. Zaffagnini S, Giordano G, Vascellari A et al (2007) Arthroscopic collagen meniscus implant results at 6–8 years follow up. Knee Surg Sports Traumatol Arthrosc 15(2):175–183
10. Bulgheroni P, Murena L, Ratti C, Bulgheroni E, Ronga M, Cherubino P (2010) Follow-up of collagen meniscus implant patients: clinical, radiological, and magnetic resonance imaging results at 5 years. Knee 17(3):224–229
11. Monllau JC, Gelber PE, Abat F et al (2011) Outcome after partial medial meniscus substitution with the collagen meniscal implant at a minimum of 10 years' follow-up. Arthroscopy 27(7):933–943
12. Burke JF (1983) Observations on the development of an artificial skin. J Trauma 23:543–551
13. Yannas IV, Orgill DP, Silver J et al (1985) Polymeric template facilitates regeneration of sciatic nerve across a 15 mm gap. Polym Mater Sci Eng 53:216–218
14. Li ST, Archibald SJ, Krarup C et al (1990) Semipermeable collagen nerve conduits for peripheral nerve regeneration. Polym Mater Sci Eng 62:575–582
15. Genovese E, Angeretti MG, Ronga M et al (2007) Follow-up of collagen meniscus implants by MRI. Radiol Med 112(7):1036–1048
16. Stone KR, Rosenberg T (1993) Surgical technique of meniscal replacement. Arthroscopy 9(2):234–237
17. Zaffagnini S, Marcheggiani Muccioli GM, Lopomo N et al (2011) Prospective long-term outcomes of the medial collagen meniscus implant versus partial meniscectomy: a minimum 10-year follow-up study. Am J Sports Med 39(5):977–985
18. Rodkey WG, DeHaven KE, Montgomery WH III et al (2008) Comparison of the collagen meniscus implant with partial meniscectomy: a prospective randomized trial. J Bone Joint Surg Am 90(7):1413–1426

Polyurethane Implant (ACTIFIT)

7

Rene Verdonk

7.1 Basic Science

Jacquelien de Groot[1]

7.1.1 Introduction

Increased awareness of potentially detrimental outcomes following partial meniscectomy led to the development of a novel meniscal scaffold, Actifit™, by Orteq Bioengineering. It received the CE Mark in July 2008 for treatment of medial or lateral irreparable partial meniscal tears. Actifit™ consists of highly interconnected porous synthetic material (Fig. 7.1) enabling tissue ingrowth. Over time, transformation into meniscus-like tissue takes place as the implant slowly degrades. Furthermore, Actifit™ is made of an aliphatic polyurethane, which provides optimal mechanical strength, biocompatibility, porosity, safe degradation and ease of use required for the indication. It is available in two shapes, medial and lateral (Fig. 7.2).

R. Verdonk (✉)
Department of Orthopaedics and Trauma, University Hospital, De Pintelaan 185, 9000 Gent, Belgium
e-mail: Rene.verdonk@ugent.be

[1] Kamerlingheplein 16, 9712 TR, Groningen, The Netherlands. e-mail: jenhde.groot@wxs.nl

R. Verdonk et al. (eds.), *Meniscal Transplantation*,
DOI: 10.1007/978-3-642-38106-5_7, © ISAKOS 2013

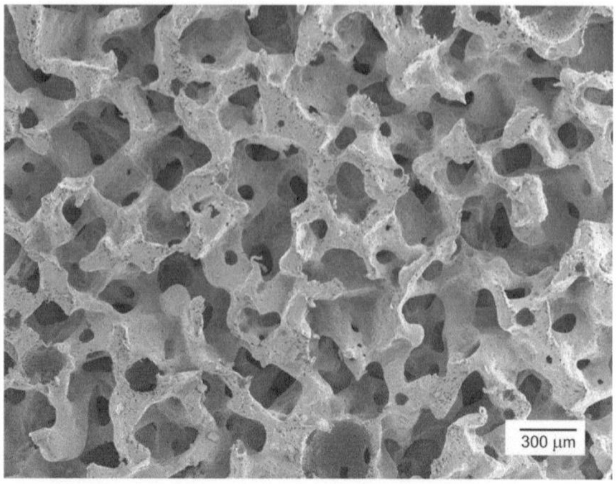

Fig. 7.1 Scanning electron micrograph of the porous structure of Actifit^{TM}

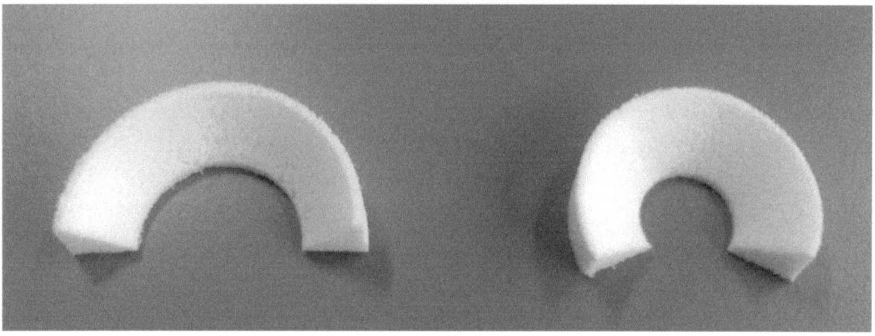

Fig. 7.2 Medial and lateral Actifit^{TM}

7.1.2 Background

Development of the meniscal scaffold started in the 1980s. Scaffold materials made of various synthetic polymers were tested in animal studies as meniscal repair or meniscal replacement material [1–22]. Based on these studies, a set of requirements for the optimal implant with respect to pore size, porosity, rate of degradation, degradation products, mechanical properties, and importantly ease of use in an arthroscopic procedure were developed. With respect to the mechanical properties, a high suture pull-out strength and sufficient stiffness became essential. Synthetic polymers currently used as biodegradable polymers for implantable devices are mainly copolymers based on lactide, ε-caprolactone, glycolide and trimethylene carbonate, and cannot fulfill all these requirements.

Polyurethanes are a class of materials with properties ranging from very brittle and hard to very tough, soft and tacky, and viscous [14]. The molecular structure can be tuned and consequently also the mechanical properties and rate of degradation. They are composed of alternating polydisperse blocks of soft and hard segments (Fig. 7.3). These qualities combined with excellent biocompatibility make polyurethanes one of the most promising synthetic biomaterials [23]. Apart from the Orteq implant, marketed polyurethanes all contain (aromatic) diisocyanate moieties, which may yield a small amount of toxic diamines upon degradation. Although it has never been proven that toxic diamines are released or that such a release would cause problems, and aromatic polyurethanes have successfully been implanted in dogs as meniscal reconstruction material in the past [1–4, 7–11, 17, 18, 20–22, 24], the possibility of toxic amine release has given polyurethanes a negative perception. Therefore, it was decided to focus on polyurethanes based on 1,4-butanediisocyanate [16, 25–33]. Upon degradation, this aliphatic polyurethane will release 1,4-butanediamine, also known as putrescine, already naturally present in the body.

7.1.3 A New Synthetic Polymer

The Actifit™ polymer consists of two components, polyester (soft segments) and polyurethane (hard segments), specifically developed and tuned for meniscal application [29]. The soft segment, 80 % of the polymer, is a biodegradable polyester, poly (ε-caprolactone). It provides flexibility and determines the degradation rate. The semi-degradable, semicrystalline, polyurethane hard segments (20 % of the polymer) are of uniform size and provide mechanical strength.

Poly (ε-caprolactone) (lines in polymer chain in Fig. 7.3) is a degradable polyester found in several implantable biodegradable medical devices, mainly sutures (Monocryl by Ethicon; Caprosyn by Tyco Healthcare) and coatings of sutures (Vicryl and Panacryl by Ethicon; Dexon and Polysorb by Tyco Healthcare). The polyurethane hard segments (white boxes in polymer chain in Fig. 7.3) contain two 1,4-butanediisocyanate (BDI) and one 1,4- butanediol (BDO) moieties and are designed to be very small (2–3 nm), i.e. approximately 5,000 times smaller than a human cell.

In order to obtain a polyurethane with excellent mechanical properties comparable to the properties of aromatic polyurethanes, the conventional polyurethane synthesis process had to be changed [25]. The polyurethane is made without a catalyst, which contributes to the polymer biocompatibility. The absence of a

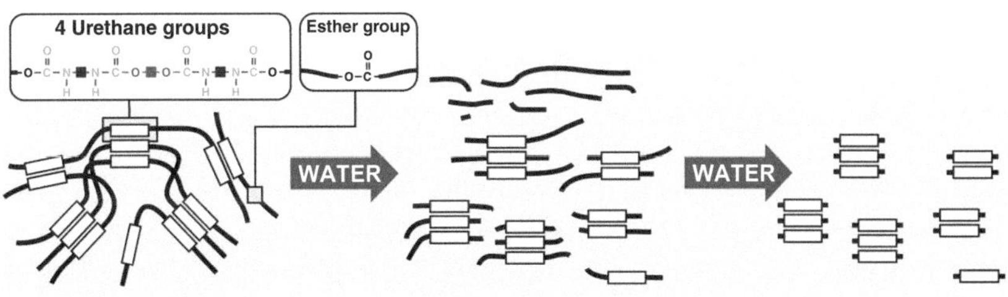

Fig. 7.3 Hydrolysis of the Actifit™ polyurethane

catalyst also contributes to the uniformity of the hard segments, and therefore to the mechanical properties of the polyurethane [29].

7.1.4 Degradation

The Actifit™ polyurethane has a very low degradation rate. The degradation mechanism takes place in the presence of water through hydrolysis of the ester bonds in the poly (ε-caprolactone) soft segments (Fig. 7.3). The polyurethane hard segments are more stable than the polycaprolactone segments and remain after hydrolysis of polycaprolactone. It is expected that these segments do not degrade in when integrated in. In case the polyurethane segments are phagocytized by macrophages (or giant cells), the hard segments degrade safely. This was determined in scientific studies of a polyurethane with similar polyurethane hard segments [34, 35] and was confirmed in Orteq's biocompatibility testing program on hard segments [36].

Degradation of the polycaprolactone segments is expected to take 4–6 years. In-vitro degradation testing (at 37 °C in phosphate buffer at pH 7.4) showed that after 1.5 years the molecular weight of the polyurethane decreased to 50 % of its original molecular weight while the implant weight was not reduced [16].

The biocompatibility of identified degradation products has either been tested by Orteq, or extensive documentation of their nontoxicity in the quantities released was already available. An overview of the tests performed is shown in the next section [37–39].

7.1.5 Preclinical Biocompatibility and Animal Testing

Orteq has completed a number of biocompatibility tests on the Actifit™ implant and on hard segments (Table 7.1). Actifit™ has passed all tests.

Two dog (beagles) studies were performed with the Actifit™ material [24, 40]. In the first study Actifit™ was implanted following total meniscectomy [24]. The follow-up period was 6 months. The implant horns were fixed on the tibial plateau with sutures pulled through drill holes in the tibia. Total meniscectomy served as control. In the second study Actifit™ was implanted for 6 and 24 weeks, with total meniscectomy and native menisci as controls [40]. The Actifit™ implants were fully integrated into the tissue without capsule formation, and the immunological response was very mild, not exceeding grade I. Histological examination of the tissue ingrowth disclosed formation of meniscus-like tissue containing proteoglycans and type II collagen (Fig. 7.4). A chondroprotective effect was not expected nor observed, due to limitations of the animal model. Nevertheless, it was hypothesized that absence of chondroprotection could be implant material-related [24]. No definite conclusions could be drawn since in this particular model the tibial plateaus were severely damaged due to technical issues in the group

Table 7.1 Tests Orteq has performed on Actifit™

Testing requirements	Relevant standards
Cytotoxicity	ISO10993-05
Sensitization	ISO10993-10
Intracutaneous irritation	ISO10993-10
Acute systemic toxicity	ISO10993-11
Combined subchronic toxicity and local tolerance (implant and hard segments)	ISO 10993-06 and ISO10993-11
Combined chronic toxicity and local tolerance (implant and hard segments)	ISO 10993-06 and ISO10993-11
Genotoxicity: bacterial reverse mutation	ISO10993-03
Genotoxicity: chromosomal aberration test in mammalian cell in vitro	ISO10993-03
Genotoxicity: mouse bone marrow micronucleus	ISO10993-03
Wear debris on small particles rabbit knee	ISO10993-06 (adapted)

receiving the implant. In a subsequent, recent sheep study Actifit™ was implanted after partial meniscectomy, with partial meniscectomy serving as control [41]. The material was found not to negatively affect the articular cartilage. In addition, the friction coefficient of the Actifit™ did not appear to be significantly different from that of native meniscus after 3 months.

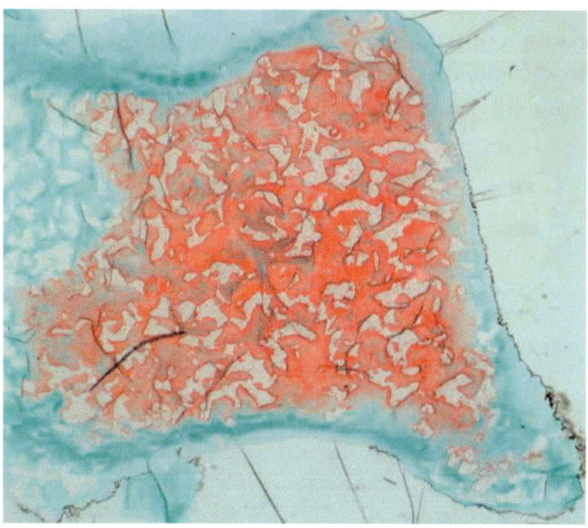

Fig. 7.4 Light micrograph of the posterior part of an Actifit™ implant, 24 months after implantation in a dog. *White areas* polymer; *green areas* fibrous tissue mainly containing type I collagen; *red areas* fibrocartilage-like tissue containing proteoglycans and mainly type II collagen

7.1.6 Clinical Results

Clinical results for Actifit™ showed significant improvement from baseline at 3, 6 and 12 months postimplantation, as evidenced by the Visual Analogue Scale (VAS), and the International Knee Documentation Committee (IKDC), Knee Injury and Osteoarthritis Outcome (KOOS) and Lysholm scores. DCMRI scans showed tissue ingrowth in 85.7 % of subjects already at 3 months postimplantation, while biopsies at 12 months showed cells with meniscus-like differentiation potential [42]. In conclusion, Actifit™ is a novel, biocompatible, polymer device specifically designed for use as a matrix for tissue ingrowth to treat irreparable meniscal defects.

7.2 Technique and Results

Rene Verdonk[2]
Peter Verdonk[3]
Eva-Lisa Heinrichs[4]

7.2.1 Introduction

Pain and other short and long-term sequelae of irreparable meniscal tears remain a challenge for the orthopedic community and there is a genuine need for an approach which will offer patients and surgeons new acceptable treatment options.

Orteq Ltd (London UK) has developed a polyurethane scaffold, Actifit®, for blood vessel ingrowth and meniscal tissue regeneration intended for the treatment of irreparable, painful meniscus tears and meniscal tissue defects. It is available in the medial and lateral configurations (Fig. 7.5). Criteria for use include an intact meniscal rim and sufficient tissue in the anterior and posterior horns to permit fixation of the scaffold. Other requirements include a well aligned and stable knee joint, an ICRS classification grade ≤ 3, a body mass index <35 kg/m^2 and the non-presence of systemic disease or infection sequelae.

[2] Department of Orthopaedics and Trauma, University Hospital, De Pintelaan 185, 9000 Gent, Belgium. e-mail: Rene.verdonk@ugent.be

[3] Department of orthopaedics and trauma, Monica ziekenhuizen, 2000 Antwerpen, Belgium.

[4] Tissue Therapies Europe Limited, Unit F34, Daresbury Innovation Centre, Keckwick Lane, Daresbury, Cheshire WA4 4FS, England. e-mail: heinrichsel@aol.com

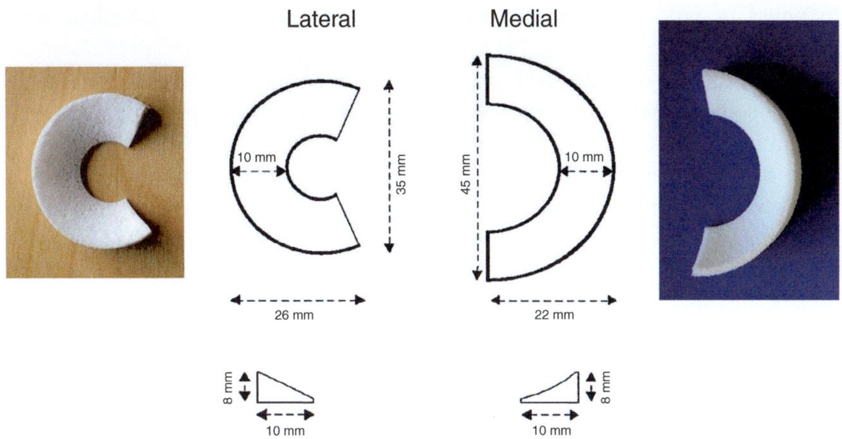

Fig. 7.5 The Actifit® meniscal scaffold comes in medial and lateral configurations

7.2.2 Implantation Procedure, Post-operative Care and Rehabilitation

7.2.2.1 Implantation Procedure

Implantation of the Actifit® meniscal scaffold is performed arthroscopically using standard surgical arthroscopic knee procedures and equipment. Detailed instructions and related warnings and precautions are set out in the Instructions for Use accompanying the device.

Using spinal or general anaesthesia at the discretion of the orthopaedic surgeon the implantation of the Actifit® meniscal scaffold is usually performed under tourniquet conditions. Thigh fixation may be used for appropriate valgus stress positioning.

Prior to implantation of either the medial and lateral scaffold, cartilage status and meniscal wall remnant status and integrity should be assessed. In the case of the lateral meniscus, meniscal wall integrity across the hiatus popliteus is essential for secure fixation and optimal tissue regeneration. All pathological cartilage and ligamentous findings should be carefully recorded.

In the case of a tight medial compartment, the medial collateral ligament (MCL) can be distended using the outside-in puncture method. Under valgus stress, and directed by the inside arthroscopic light, the surgeon is able to bring a needle in the posteromedial side of the knee joint into joint. The MCL is sensed and allows for progressive pie-crusting of the ligament until the appropriate opening is obtained.

The inside-out pie crusting release technique as described by Steadman can also be used. Under arthroscopic control, the posteromedial corner of the knee joint is visualised. Using the Steadman pick, the MCL can be reached and progressively disrupted in order to open the knee joint appropriately until visualisation is obtained.

In the lateral compartment progressive pie-crusting release techniques as described above and used in the medial compartment are not possible because of anatomical considerations; however, lateral compartment narrowing is rare.

To facilitate healing, the meniscal rim can be punctured for vascular access channels and gentle rasping of the synovial lining is recommended. After debridement and preparation, the defect should reach into the red–red or red-white zone, approximately 1–2 mm from the synovial border. The defect should thereafter be measured along its inner margin using the meniscal ruler and meniscal ruler guide which accompany the Actifit® device.

The Actifit® meniscal scaffold should be measured and cut using a scalpel (Fig. 7.6). Sterility should be continually maintained. Care should be taken not to undersize the device. For the purpose of achieving a snug fit into the defect, the length of the scaffold should be oversized by approximately 10 %, i.e. 3 mm for small defects (<3 cm) and approximately 5 mm for large defects (≥3 cm). It is recommended that the anterior side be cut at an angle of 30–45° for easier suturing (Fig. 7.7).

For the implantation 2–3 small incisions for anteromedial and anterolateral portals are needed. An arthroscopic central transpatellar tendon portal is optional. For easy insertion of the scaffold, we recommend that the relevant portal is sized sufficiently to approximately the size of the little finger. In addition, a posteromedial or posterolateral incision may be required if an inside-out meniscal fixation technique is used.

Although the Actifit® material is easy to manipulate and is strong and flexible, it should be handled with care. The tailored Actifit® scaffold can be introduced into the knee joint through the anteromedial or anterolateral portal using a non cannulated tissue tension grasper such as the Acuflex Grasper Tissue Tensioner™ (Smith and Nephew) (Fig. 7.8). Marking the cranial and caudal scaffold surface

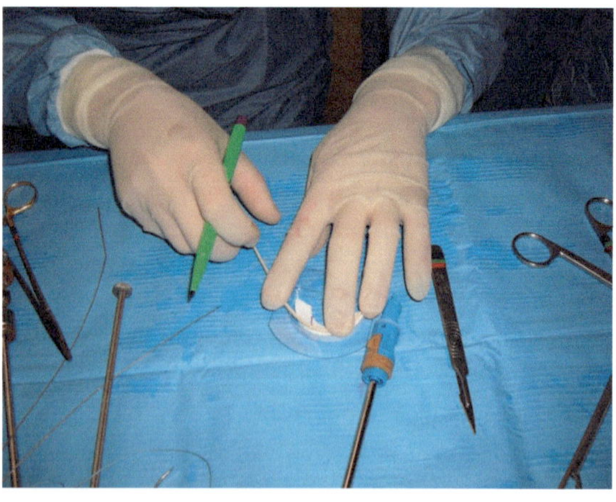

Fig. 7.6 The Actifit meniscal scaffold is tailored using a scalpel for a snug fit to the meniscus defect

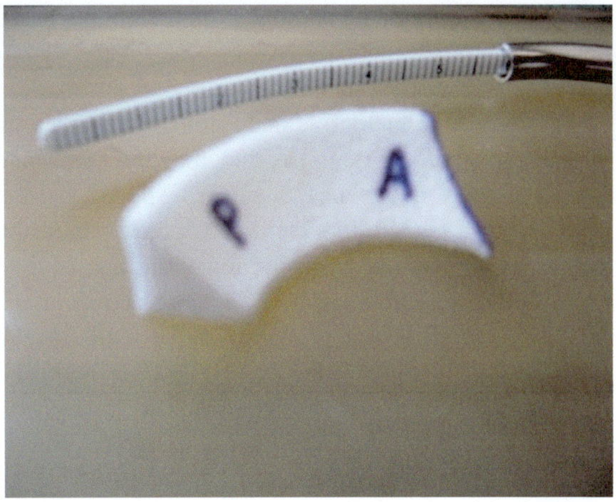

Fig. 7.7 The anterior side should cut at an angle of 30–45° for easier suturing

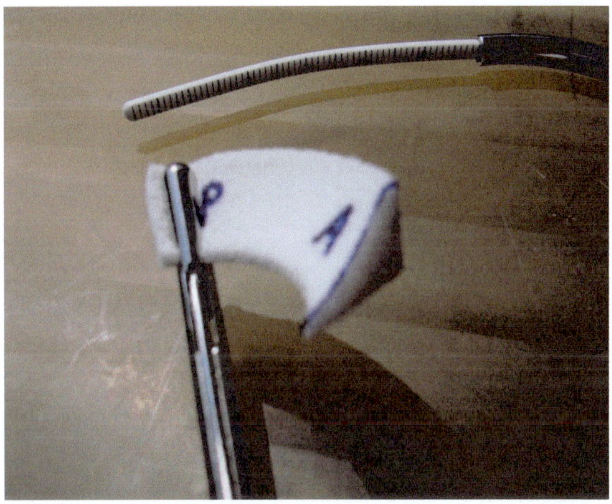

Fig. 7.8 The scaffold device should be manipulated using a blunt nose grasper. It is useful to mark the cranial and caudal meniscal scaffold surface

helps to avoid problems in positioning. The Actifit® scaffold should be clamped at the posterior part of the scaffold and placed into the knee joint through the anteromedial or anterolateral portal. To ensure a good initial position of the scaffold and facilitate fixation, a vertical holding suture may be placed in the native mensicus tissue to bring the scaffold through the eye of this holding suture.

Fixation of Actifit® is accomplished by suturing the scaffold to the native meniscus tissue. Standard commercially available size 2.0 non-resorbable sutures, such as polyester or polypropylene and braided or monofil sutures are recommended. Which suturing techniques are used depends on the location of the defect and the surgeon's experience and preference. All-inside suturing is commonly used for the posterior horn and posterior part of the rim. All-inside, inside-out and outside-in techniques may be used for the middle and anterior part of the rim.

Horizontal sutures with an outside-in technique are commonly used for the anterior horn.

Fixation should start with a horizontal all-inside suture from the posterior edge of the scaffold to the native meniscus. Suturing should be secure; however, sutures must not be over-tightened as they may alter and indent the surface of the scaffold. The distances between the sutures should be kept to approximately 0.5 cm (Fig. 7.9a). Each suture should be placed at one-third to one-half of the scaffold's height, as determined from the lower surface of the scaffold (Fig. 7.9b). Suturing through the musculus popliteus are not detrimental to later function.

Once sutured in place if required, the scaffold may be further trimmed and fine-tuned intra-articularly using a basket punch. Stability of the fixation is tested using the probe and carefully moving the knee through a range of motion (0–90°).

7.2.2.2 Post Operative Care

Following implantation of the Actifit® scaffold, pain and thromboprophylactic medications are administered at the surgeon's discretion and would be those typically administered following classic meniscal suturing.

Dependent upon the meniscal scaffold stability as determined at the end of the surgical procedure, a rigid removable brace may be used over a compression bandage in the first week post-implantation.

7.2.2.3 Post Operative Rehabilitation

Following implantation of the Actifit® scaffold the recommended post operative rehabilitation protocol should be strictly followed to ensure optimum conditions for healing and to protect the newly formed fragile tissue from potentially harmful stresses whilst tissue remodelling and maturation processes are ongoing during the

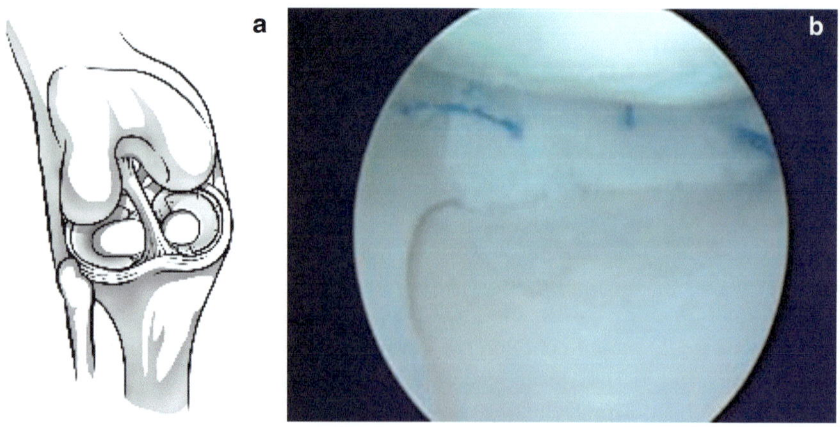

Fig. 7.9 **a** The distances between the sutures should approximately 0.5 cm. **b** Each suture should be placed at one-third to one-half of the scaffold height determined from the lower surface of the scaffold in order to allow proper fixation

first 3 months post-surgery. It is important that the rehabilitation protocol is reviewed and approved to be suitable for the patient in question by the responsible orthopaedic surgeon and carried out under the supervision of a professional physiotherapist.

Non weight-bearing is recommended until 4 weeks post-surgery. Partial weight bearing is permitted from 4 weeks onward with a gradual increase in loading up to 100 % load at 9 weeks post-implantation, at a rate of 10 kg per week for patients weighing ≤60 kg and 15 kg per week for patients weighing ≤90 kg, and without the use of the unloader brace from week 14 onwards.

Under the rehabilitation protocol, motion is initiated immediately after implantation, with bending up to 30° with full extension permitted in weeks 1 and 2. Flexion is increased to 60° in week 3, and to 90° in weeks 4 and 5. From week 6 onwards, flexion is further increased until a full range of motion is achieved; however, forceful movements should be avoided. Light exercise, including isometric quadricps exercises, mobilsation of the patella, heel slides, quad sets, anti-equinus foot exercises and Achilles tendon stretching, is advised from week 1. As of 9 weeks, additional exercises, including increased closed hamstring exercises, lunges between 0 and 90°, proprioception exercises, dynamic quadriceps expercises and use of a home trainer, are indicated. Increased open and closed exercises, jogging on level ground, plyometris and sports-related exercises without pivot are recommended from week 14 onwards. Hydrotherapy and swimming (crawl and headstroke) can commence 24 weeks post-implantation. Gradual resumption of other sports is generally commenced as of 6 months at the discretion of the responsible orthopaedic surgeon; however, contact sports should be resumed only after 9 months.

7.2.3 Clinical Results

Safety, performance and efficacy results to support use of the Actifit® scaffold in the treatment of painful irreparable meniscal defects were obtained from a prospective, non-randomised, single-arm, clinical investigation conducted at 9 orthopaedic centres of excellence located throughout Europe. Patients recruited (N = 52) had an irreparable medial or lateral meniscus tear or partial meniscus loss, intact rim, presence of both horns and a stable well-aligned knee.

Thirty-four patients were treated with a medial meniscal scaffold and 18 patients were treated with a lateral meniscal scaffold. Demographics and baseline characteristics were representative of the population for which Actifit® is intended. The mean patient age was 30.8 ± 9.4 years and 75 % were male. The mean longitudinal defect length was 47.1 ± 10.0 mm.

The study follow-up period was 24 months and the study has been reported in the American Journal of Sports Medicine [43].

7.3 Safety Results

Nine index knee-related Serious Adverse Events (SAEs) were reported in the study (five in the medial and four in the lateral indication. Three of these in the medial indication and three in the lateral indication resulted in withdrawal. Four of the nine SAEs were reported as unrelated to the scaffold and to the procedure; four were reported as procedure related; none were reported as having a definite, probable, or possible relationship to the Actifit® scaffold.

One SAE was reported as having an unknown relationship to the Actifit® scaffold and to the procedure. This was the removal of an almost completely nonintegrated scaffold, which took place at the protocol stipulated relook arthroscopy. The patient was asymptomatic and importantly no signs of inflammatory reaction to the scaffold and no evidence of cartilage damage were observed during gross examination. A biopsy specimen taken from the meniscus rim post removal of the nonintegrated scaffold material showed cell-populated scaffold material integrated with tissue. No inflammatory reaction to the scaffold was observed in the biopsy. It was concluded that the integration failure was most likely due to lack of biological response.

Cartilage scores in the index compartment were assessed at 3, 12 and 24 months post-implantation using anatomic MRI scans. Stable or improved cartilage status at 24 months was demonstrated in 92.5 % (37/40) of patients compared with baseline status.

7.3.1 Efficacy Results

Pain and functionality were assessed using validated clinical outcome scores. The Visual Analog Scale (VAS), was used for knee pain, at 3, 6, 12 and 24 months post-implantation. The International Knee Documentation Committee (IKDC), the Lysholm score, as well as the Knee and Osteoarthritis Outcome Score (KOOS) were used to assess functionality.

For functionality on IKDC and Lysholm scores and for pain (VAS), statistically and clinically significant improvements from baseline to 24 months were reported at 3, 6, 12 and 24 months post implantation ($p < 0.05$).

Statistically and clinically significant improvements ($p < 0.05$) were also reported for the five KOOS subcomponents: for pain, activities of daily living and quality of life at 3, 6, 12 and 24 months, and for sports/recreation and symptoms at 6, 12 and 24 months post implantation.

7.3.2 Evidence of New Tissue Formation

Tissue ingrowth into the Actifit® scaffold was assessed during the protocol stipulated relook arthroscopy at 12 months ($n = 44$) by gross examination and histological examination of biopsies from the inner free edge of the implanted scaffold.

Presence of vital tissue with no necrosis or cell death and hence consistent with biocompatibility of the scaffold was observed in all 44 biopsies at 12 months. Moreover, the histology data suggested an ongoing process of regeneration, remodelling and maturation towards tissue resembling the human meniscus.

Tissue ingrowth was also assessed at 3 months post-implantation by evidence of vascularisation in the scaffold using diagnostic contrast enhanced MRI (DCE-MRI) (n = 43). All scans were assessed for neovascularisation in the peripheral half of the scaffold meniscus.

At 3 months post-implantation, early evidence of tissue ingrowth was observed on DCE-MRI in the peripheral half of the scaffold, in 35 of 43 (81.4 %) patients.

7.3.3 Conclusion

No safety concerns, other than those generally acknowledged with this type of surgery, were identified. Importantly, no safety issues related to the device, including cartilage damage or inflammatory reaction to the Actifit® scaffold or its degradation products, were observed. Efficacy data showed significant (statistical and clinical) improvement from pre-operative status for the subjective clinical outcome scores as of 3–24 months post-implantation. The 24-month clinical results provide strong evidence of the safety and efficacy of the Actifit® scaffold treatment option for a patient group for whom currently only restricted treatment options are available. In addition, compared to partial meniscectomy, treatment of irreparable meniscus defects with the Actifit® scaffold has the benefit of promoting new tissue generation.

References

1. Elema H, de Groot JH, Nijenhuis AJ, Pennings AJ, Veth RPH, Klompmaker J, Jansen HWB (1990) Use of biodegradable polymer implants in meniscus reconstruction: 2 biological evaluation of porous biodegradable implants in menisci. Colloid Polym Sci 268:1082–1088
2. de Groot JH (1995) Porous polymeric elastomers for repair and replacement of the knee joint meniscus. PhD thesis, State University Groningen, The Netherlands. http://dissertations.ub.rug.nl/FILES/faculties/science/1995/j.h.de.groot/titlecon.pdf
3. de Groot JH, Nijenhuis AJ, Bruin P, Pennings AJ, Veth RPH, Klompmaker J, Jansen HWB (1990) Use of biodegradable polymer implants in meniscus reconstruction. 1 Preparation of porous biodegradable polyurethanes for the reconstruction of the meniscus. Colloid Polym Sci 268:1073–1081
4. de Groot JH, de Vrijer R, Pennings AJ, Klompmaker J, Veth RPH, Jansen HWB (1996) Use of porous polyurethanes for meniscal reconstruction and prosthesis. Biomaterials 17:163–173
5. de Groot JH, Zijlstra FM, Kuipers HW, Pennings AJ, Klompmaker J, Veth RPH, Jansen HWB (1997) Meniscal tissue regeneration in porous 50/50 copoly (L-lactide/ε-caprolactone) implants. Biomaterials 18:613–622
6. de Groot JH, Kuiper HW, Pennings AJ (1997) A novel method for fabrication biodegradable scaffolds with high compression moduli. J Mater Sci Mater Med 8:703

7. Heijkants RG, van Calck RV, van Tienen TG, de Groot JH, Pennings AJ, Buma P, Veth RP, Schouten AJ (2008) Polyurethane scaffold formation via a combination of salt leaching and thermally induced phase separation. J Biomed Mater Res A 15(87):921–932
8. Klompmaker J (1992) Porous polymers for repair and replacement of the knee joint meniscus and articualr cartilage. PhD thesis, State University Groningen, The Netherlands
9. Klompmaker J, Jansen HWB, Veth RPH, de Groot JH, Nijenhuis AJ, Pennings AJ (1991) Porous polymer implants for repair of meniscal lesions: a preliminary study in dogs. Biomaterials 12:810–816
10. Klompmaker J, Jansen HWB, Veth RPH, de Groot JH, Penings Kuijer R (1992) Meniscal repair by fibrocartilage: An experimental study in the dog. J Orthop Res 10:359–370
11. Klompmaker J, Jansen HWB, Veth RPH, de Groot JH, Nijenhuis AJ, Pennings AJ (1992) Porous polymer implants for repair of full-thickness defects of articular cartilage: an experimental study in the dog. Biomaterials 13:625–634
12. Klompmaker J, Jansen HWB, Veth RPH, Nielsen HKL, de Groot JH, Pennings AJ (1994) Porous implants for the knee joint meniscus reconstruction: A preliminary study on the role of pore sizes in ingrowth and differentiation of fibrocartilage. Clin Mater 14:1–11
13. Klompmaker J, Jansen HWB, Veth RPH, Nielsen NKL, de Groot JH, Pennings AJ (1996) Meniscal replacement using a porous polymer prosthesis: a preliminary study in the dog. Bimoaterials 17:1169–1176
14. Lamba NMK, Woodhouse KA, Cooper SL (1998) Polyurethanes in Biomedical Applications. CRC press, Boca Raton
15. Leenslag JW (1987) Poly (L-lactide) and its biomedical applications. PhD thesis, State University Groningen, The Netherlands
16. Orteq report R08006 in vitro degradation study Actifit™
17. Spaans CJ, de Groot JH, Dekens FG, Veth RPH, Pennings AJ (1999) Development of new polyurethanes for repair and replacement of the knee joint meniscus. Polym Prep 40:589–590
18. Spaans CJ, Belgraver VW, Rienstra OR, Veth RPH, de Groot JH, Pennings AJ (2000) Solvent-free fabrication of micro-porous polyurethane amide and polyurethane urea scaffolds for repair and replacement of the knee joint meniscus. Biomaterials 21:2453–2460
19. van Tienen TG (2004) In-vivo tissue engineering of knee joint meniscus. PhD thesis, University Nijmegen, The Netherlands
20. van Tienen TG, Heijkants RG, Buma P, de Groot JH, Pennings AJ, Veth RP (2002) Tissue ingrowth and degradation of two biodegradable porous polymers with different porosities and pore sizes. Biomaterials 23:1731–1738
21. van Tienen TG, Heijkants RG, de Groot JH, Pennings AJ, Poole AR, Veth RP, Buma P (2003) Presence and mechanism of knee articular cartilage degeneration after meniscal reconstruction in dogs. Osteoarthritis Cartilage 11:78–84
22. Tienen TG, Heijkants RG, de Groot JH, Schouten AJ, Pennings AJ, Veth RP, Buma P (2006) Meniscal replacement in dogs. Tissue regeneration in two different materials with similar properties. J Biomed Mater Res B Appl Biomater 76:389–396
23. Klompmaker J, Jansen HWB, Veth PRH, Nielsen NKL, de Groot JH, Pennings AJ, Kuijer R (1996) Meniscal repair by fibrocartilage in the dog: Characterization of the repair tissue and the role of vascularity. Biomaterials 17:1685–1692
24. van Tienen TG, Heijkants RG, Buma P, de Groot JH, Pennings AJ, Veth RP (2003) A porous polymer scaffold for meniscal lesion repair: A study in dogs. Biomaterials 24:2541–2548
25. de Groot JH, de Vrijer R, Wildeboer BS, Spaans CJ, Pennings AJ (1997) New biomedical polyurethane ureas with high tear strength. Polym Bull 38:211–218
26. de Groot JH, Spaans CJ, Dekens FG, Pennings AJ (1998) On the role of aminolysis and transesterification in the synthesis of ε-caprolactone and L-lactide based polyurethanes. Polym Bull 41:299–306
27. Heijkants RGJC (2004) Polyurethane scaffolds as meniscus reconstruction material. PhD thesis, State University Groningen, The Netherlands. http://dissertations.ub.rug.nl/faculties/science/2004/r.g.j.c.heijkants/

28. Heijkants RG, van Calck RV, De Groot JH, Pennings AJ, Schouten AJ, van Tienen TG, Ramrattan N, Buma P, Veth RP (2004) Design, synthesis and properties of a degradable polyurethane scaffold for meniscus regeneration. J Mater Sci Mater Med 15:423–427
29. Heijkants RG, van Calck RV, van Tienen TG, de Groot JH, Buma P, Pennings AJ, Veth RP, Schouten AJ (2005) Uncatalyzed synthesis, thermal and mechanical properties of polyurethanes based on poly(epsilon-caprolactone) and 1,4-butane diisocyanate with uniform hard segment. Biomaterials 26:4219–4228
30. Orteq report R06036(2) Summary Biocompatibility Testing Actifit™
31. Ramrattan NN, Heijkants RG, van Tienen TG, Schouten AJ, Veth RP, Buma P (2005) Assessment of tissue ingrowth rates in polyurethane scaffolds for tissue engineering. Tissue Eng 11:1212–1223
32. Spaans CJ (2000) Biomedical polyurethanes based on 1,4-butanediisocyanate. PhD thesis, State University Groningen, The Netherlands
33. Spaans CJ, de Groot JH, Dekens FG, Pennings AJ (1998) High molecular weight polyurethanes and a polyurethane urea based on 1,4-butanediisocyanate. Polym Bull 41:131–138
34. Maher SA, Doty SB, Rodeo SA, Brophy R, Potter H, Foo L, Rosenblatt L, Deng X-H, Turner AS, Wright TM, Warren RF. Evaluation of a Porous Polyurethane Scaffold in a partial meniscal defect ovine model. To be published
35. Veth RP, Jansen HW, Leenslag JW, Pennings AJ, Hartel RM, Nielsen HK (1986) Experimental meniscal lesions reconstructed with a carbon fiber-polyurethane-poly (L-lactide) graft. Clin Orthop Relat Res 202:286–293
36. van Minnen B, van Leeuwen MB, Kors G, Zuidema J, van Kooten TG, Bos RR (2008) In vivo resorption of a biodegradable polyurethane foam, based on 1,4-butanediisocyanate: a three-year subcutaneous implantation study. J Biomed Mater Res A 15(85):972–982
37. Spaans CJ, Belgraver VW, de Groot JH, Pennings AJ (1998) A new biomedical polyurethane with a high modulus based on 1,4-butanediisocyanate. J Mater Sci Mater Med 9:675–678
38. Welsing RT, van Tienen TG, Ramrattan N, Heijkants R, Schouten AJ, Veth RP, Buma P (2008) Effect on tissue differentiation and articular cartilage degradation of a polymer meniscus implant: A 2-year follow-up study in dogs. Am J Sports Med 36:1978 1989
39. Zuidema J, van Minnen B, Span MM, Hissink CE, van Kooten TG, Bos RR (2008) In vitro degradation of a biodegradable polyurethane foam, based on 1,4-butanediisocyanate: A 3-year study at physiological and elevated temperature. J Biomed Mater Res A (Epub ahead of print)
40. Verdonk P, Verdonk R on behalf of the Actifit Study Group (2009) Clinical efficacy and safety of a resorbable meniscus scaffold for the treatment of partial meniscal tear or meniscal loss. International Meeting on Early Intervention for Knee Arthritis, Maastricht 4–6 February 2009
41. Leenslag JW, Nijenhuis AJ, Pennings AJ, Veth RPH, Nielsen HKL, Jansen HWB (1986) Porous composites for repair of the meniscus. Proceedings of the P.I.M.S V, Noordwijkerhout, The Netherlands, 10–12 September, pp 10/1–10/9
42. Tienen TG, Heijkants RG, de Groot JH, Pennings AJ, Schouten AJ, Veth RP, Buma P (2006) Replacement of the knee meniscus by a porous polymer implant: a study in dogs. Am J Sports Med 34:64–71
43. Verdonk P, Beaufils P, Bellemans J, Djian P, Heinrichs EL, Huysse W, Laprell H, Siebold R, Verdonk R, Actifit Study Group (2012) Successful treatment of painful irreparable partial meniscal defects with a polyurethane scaffold: two-year safety and clinical outcomes. Am J Sports Med 40(4):844–853 (Epub 2012 Feb 9)

8 Synthesis

R. Verdonk

Clinicians are more confronted with issues dealing with partial meniscectomy and functional derangement.

In animal experiments, collagen meniscus implantation (CMI) was found to yield good results and function. The regenerated tissue appeared to be similar to the native meniscus. The implants did not induce degenerative changes, abrasion or synovitis, and were devoid of allergic or immune responses.

Human clinical trials, which were conducted at various centres over longer periods of time, showed a lesser need for revision surgery after CMI implantation in chronic meniscectomized knees, compared to controls.

Good alignment and stability are preoperative requirements.

Alternatives were searched for that would allow to work with stronger as well as resorbable materials.

In animal studies, long-term assessment of a polyurethane scaffold showed that transformation into meniscus- like tissue took place as the implant slowly degraded.

Another requirement is the possibility to insert and manipulate the implant into position with use of arthroscopic techniques. A first human safety and efficacy study of 52 patients demonstrated a statistically significant improvement in quality of life and clinical scores at one year, suggesting that the implant was safe and effective.

Finally, meniscal allografts seem to sustain the hypothesis that meniscal replacement after total meniscectomy is a valid alternative, more specifically in the lateral compartment. For the medial compartment, other useful options are available.

R. Verdonk (✉)
Department of Orthopaedics and Trauma, University Hospital, De Pintelaan 185, 9000 Ghent, Belgium
e-mail: Rene.verdonk@ugent.be

R. Verdonk et al. (eds.), *Meniscal Transplantation*,
DOI: 10.1007/978-3-642-38106-5_8, © ISAKOS 2013

The more common knee dysfunction after partial meniscectomy does not warrant total meniscal allograft replacement.

While we are still constantly searching for useful modes of treatment, partial meniscal replacement is already a first step in the right direction.

Part III
The Future

Future Trends in the Treatment of Meniscus Lesions: From Repair to Regeneration

9

H. Pereira, J. Silva-Correia, J. M. Oliveira, R. L. Reis and J. Espregueira-Mendes

9.1 Introduction

"Nothing has changed so much in knee treatment and surgery as meniscal treatment algorithms"—This statement from Verdonk [1] condenses the overturn occurred in recent years concerning the approach of meniscus lesions.

The advent of tissue engineering (TE) promise to revolutionize the concept of medicine by means of using regenerative principles emerging from engineering and life sciences, to fabricate functional substitutes to restore, maintain, or improve tissue function. To achieve this goal, it makes use of three main variables, i.e., scaffolds, cells (differentiated or undifferentiated) and bioactive agents or growth factors (GFs) which can be placed into the injury zone, alone or in combination. On the other hand, regenerative medicine is a wider concept and besides comprising the use of soluble molecules and stem cell technology, it can also apply tissue engineering, nanotechnology and gene therapy strategies to restore or establish cells/tissues/organs normal functions.

The biological characterization of meniscus tissue, although not yet completely accomplished, has evolved significantly in the last few years [2, 3]. This is true concerning recognition of different cellular populations, understanding its

H. Pereira (✉) · J. Silva-Correia · J. M. Oliveira · R. L. Reis · J. Espregueira-Mendes
3B's Research Group-Biomaterials, Biodegradables and Biomimetics,
Department of Polymer Engineering, University of Minho, Guimarães, Portugal
e-mail: heldermdpereira@gmail.com

J. Espregueira-Mendes
e-mail: jem@espregueira.com

H. Pereira · J. Silva-Correia · J. M. Oliveira · R. L. Reis · J. Espregueira-Mendes
Headquarters of the European Institute of Excellence on Tissue Engineering and Regenerative Medicine, S. Cláudio do Barco, AvePark, Caldas das Taipas, 4806-909, Guimarães, Portugal

R. Verdonk et al. (eds.), *Meniscal Transplantation*,
DOI: 10.1007/978-3-642-38106-5_9, © ISAKOS 2013

ultra-structure [2], cells and extracellular matrix segmental distributions. Other important gained knowledge is related to biomechanical properties, biologic interactions or injury response mechanisms namely on relevant aspects of tissue healing/failure such as vascularization and re-innervation [2, 3].

The need for meniscal repair/regeneration is increasingly appreciated [4]. When repair is no longer possible, substitution seems to be suitable approach [5], i.e. there is a consensus in respect to total meniscus allograft transplantation in selected cases. Moreover, meniscus lesions, in its various forms, subsists as one of the most frequent injuries leading to orthopedic surgery [6]. Long term deleterious effects of meniscectomy have been reported determining functional limitation and early osteoarthritis [7]. Bearing in mind the huge socioeconomic impact of meniscus lesions, it became clear that new effective strategies [8] should be developed. TE and Regenerative Medicine has been one of the most relevant fields of research aiming to find such answers.

Within this chapter we aim to summarize relevant information in order to facilitate translating research from bench to bedside and helping the orthopedic clinician-scientists [8] in designing projects and research directions.

9.2 The 3R's: Replacement, Repair, and Regeneration

Replacement of meniscus can be both total and partial [9]. Partial replacement using meniscus cadaveric allograft transplantation (MAT) has evolved a lot since Milachowski's report [10]. A recent meta-analysis reported consistent satisfactory outcome with restoration of working capacity in active patients after MAT [5]. The complication and failure rates were considered as acceptable [5]. Meniscal allograft transplantation can be considered as safe and reliable for the treatment of refractory post-meniscectomy symptoms in selected patients [5, 11]. However, several problems should be considered in MAT such as grafts availability; managing and storage preserving biomechanical and biologic properties while preventing disease transmission; matching size and shape according to host [9].

When menisci repair is not possible, partial resection of the meniscus is an option [12]. Repair ability of meniscus is mainly related to fibrovascular scar proliferation, and the healing prognosis is dictated by location of the lesion, i.e. red–red, red–white and white–white regions [12]. The first reported surgical human meniscus repair occurred in 1885 [13]. Since then numerous repair techniques were developed, but suture repair seems to provide superior biomechanical stability [14]. Biologic factors might be of greater importance to the success of meniscus repair as compared to surgical approaches [12]. Therefore, the decision on the most appropriate repair technique should not rely on biomechanical parameters alone [14].

Meniscus repair is possible and reproducible; however up to 24 % of global failure rate has been described [15], particularly in high level athletes. Whereas meniscus repairs have higher re-operation rates than partial meniscectomies, they are associated with better long-term outcomes [16]. Besides the previous, an overall healing rate after repair has shown around 60 % of complete healing, 20 % of partial healing and 20 % had not healed on 2nd look arthroscopy [16]. Furthermore, partial meniscectomy has lower re-operation rate than menisci repair. Re-operation rates are higher after partial lateral meniscectomy compared with the medial meniscectomy. Repair of the lateral meniscus has a lower re-operation rate than repair of the medial meniscus. These data should be taken into account within therapeutic decision [16]. The repair of a meniscus lesions should always be kept in mind if the tear is peripheral and longitudinal, with concurrent anterior cruciate ligament reconstruction, particular in younger patients [14]. On the other hand, the probability of healing is decreased in complex or degenerative tears, central tears, and tears in unstable knees. Age or extension of the tear into the avascular area should not be considered exclusion criteria [14]. In opposition to repair strategies, regeneration strategies are aimed to promote formation of new tissue that likely has similar biological and biomechanical performance to native meniscus. In respect to tissue engineering regenerative strategies aiming to enhance suture repair,

Vertical tears with posterior root involvement do cause changes in joint contact pressure and area in both the medial and lateral compartments of the knee. Repair of the vertical tear reverses these contact changes, resulting in contact pressure and area similar to the intact state [17].

Contemporary all-inside repair systems have decreased the operating time and the level of surgical skill required. Despite the ease of use, there is a potential for complications because of the close proximity of vessels, nerves, and tendons [14].

TE and regenerative augmentation is a promising and ongoing field of research but, so far, has not reached effective clinical application [12].

The possibility of meniscus regeneration has also been the basis for the ongoing development of partial replacement approaches for the treatment of irreparable, painful, partial meniscus defects [12, 18]. All clinical studies so far refer to acellular scaffolds alone (collagen or polyurethane-based) [12].

For the aforementioned, the possibility of future tissue engineered implant mimicking the native tissue can provide a valuable option, thus avoiding current limitations and presenting a more favorable cost-benefit profile while improving results and lowering failure rates [12]. Figure 9.1 summarizes the perspective of *status quo* and future trends in meniscus treatment strategies based in the analysis of clinical and pre-clinical studies [12].

9.3 Advanced Regenerative Strategies

9.3.1 Tissue Engineering for Regeneration of Meniscus Lesions

9.3.1.1 Acellular Strategies Using Scaffolds

Only acellular scaffolds have been tried in clinical setting for meniscus partial replacement [12, 18]. Most studies have reported on collagen-based implants (CMI, currently known as Menaflex®, ReGen Biologics, USA) enrolling several hundred of patients, mainly for medial meniscus defects [19–26] but recently also for lateral meniscus [27].

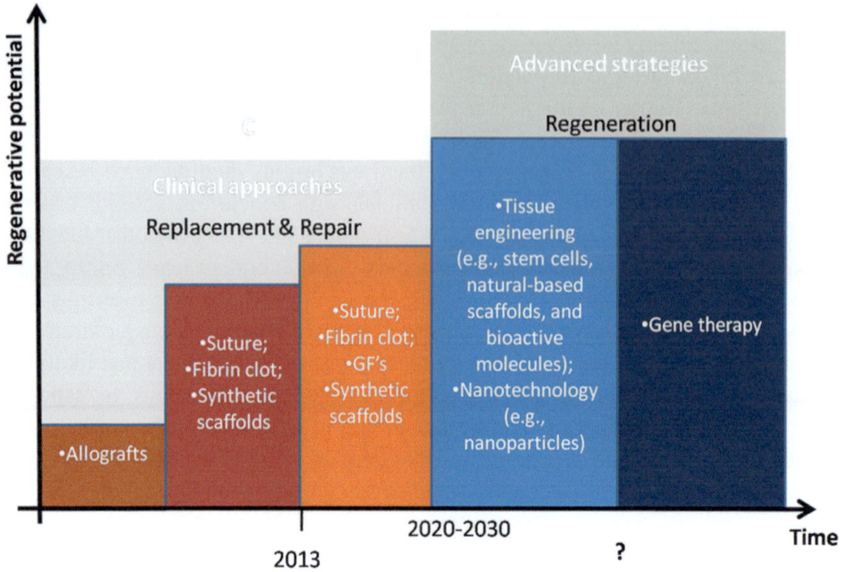

Fig. 9.1 Illustration of the different regenerative potential of the current clinical and advanced pre-clinical strategies for treatment of meniscus lesions. Expected future trends in this field

Reduced implant size with time was reported assessed by MRI or second look arthroscopy. The exact incidence of this fact has not been possible to clarify neither its magnitude nor influence in the outcome. No clinically relevant data on severe inflammation or immune response was found in any of the biopsy specimens reported [12]. Furthermore the final tissue obtained has been different than the original meniscal fibrocartilage [12]. Some concerns about initial lower mechanical properties of this biomaterial have been reported [21]. This highlights the need to further improve/augment these acellular strategies by using more complex tissue engineering strategies.

The other implant clinically tested is polyurethane-based (Actifit®, Orteq Ltd, London, United Kingdom). It has been proven that allows tissue ingrowths' [28] and it is clinically effective in cases of pain associated to irreparable partial meniscus lesions [18, 29].

However histology also demonstrates that final tissue obtained to be different than normal one and little is known about the pattern of re-cellularization [12].

Several other biomaterials are being developed and have been proposed aiming to constitute advantageous options for acellular and/or cell based strategies, including: silk fibroin [30], hyaluronic acid-polycaprolactone [31], polycaprolactone-polyurethane [32], and polyglycolic acid [33]. All of the previous studies still lack clinical validation.

A crucial aspect on the preparation of TE scaffolds is the ability to reproduce the architectural and geometric intricacies of the envisaged tissue/organ. The traditional technologies to produce scaffolds are limited to randomly control of individual pore geometry, size, interconnectivity and morphology. In past few years, solid free-form fabrication (SFF) technologies emerged as powerful methods to prepare highly organized 3D porous scaffolds as it possibly uses computer-based medical imaging technologies (e.g., CT scans or magnetic resonance imaging) to design and fabricate customized and anatomically adapted scaffolds [34]. In future, 3D fiber-deposited (3DF) anatomical scaffolds will be produced by rapid prototyping [35] after acquiring CT and MRI of the patient, and then. These will be developed with a similar shape and dimensions and with suitable mechanical behavior. The 3DSF anatomical scaffolds can be designed and fabricated with a variable, interconnected and accessible porous network, resulting in tailorable mechanical properties, permeability, and architecture that can be tuned to mimic meniscus native architecture (Fig. 9.2).

9.3.1.2 Cellular Strategies and or Bioactive Agents

A recent systematic review of TE approaches to meniscus treatment demonstrated a discrepancy between clinical trials and pre-clinical studies. While most clinical applications concern acellular strategies, most pre-clinical authors favor cells and/or bioactive agents' augmentation aiming to improve results.

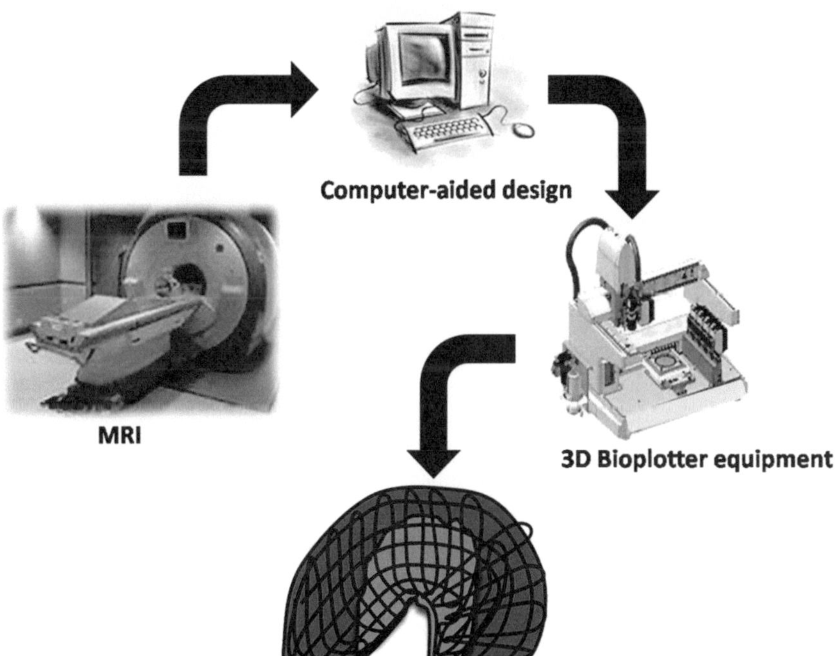

Fig. 9.2 Scheme of the fabrication of the 3D fiber-deposited (3DF) anatomical scaffolds, after acquiring CT/MRI of the patients' meniscus

Pre-clinical cell seeded scaffold approach [31, 33, 36–42] has been described. The combination of cells, scaffold and growth factors (GFs) [43, 44] sometimes adding gene therapy has also been tried [43]. Additionally, one study compared cell seeded scaffold and scaffold-GFs approaches [45] and another tested in vivo the immuno compatibility of a scaffold (decellularized porcine meniscus) but intends for a cell seeded construct approach [46]. Some authors propose the combination of scaffolds and GFs [47–49].

Martinek et al. [40] using collagen based meniscus implant for partial replacement concluded that constructs with autologous fibrochondrocytes perform better than Collagen Meniscus Implant alone. In the same stream, Angele et al. [36] found that hyaluronan/gelatin composite scaffold seeded with stem cells do better than empty scaffolds and represent a valuable possibility aiming repair of meniscus defects. Weinand et al. [41, 42] presents an implantable biodegradable construct consisting of woven vicryl mesh seeded with either allogeneic [42] or autologous [41] chondrocytes from different tissues (articular, auricular or costal). In their work [42], the authors hypothesize that combining a scaffold with cells would favor suture of meniscus lesions in avascular zone. The authors further concluded that presence of both autologous and allogeneic chondrocytes enhance meniscal healing [41], in a swine model.

A different approach aims to enhance scaffolds associating to GFs. Ishida et al. [47] reported that combining gelatin hydrogel with PRP as carrier increased healing of meniscus defects comparing to either of them isolated.

Considering the TERM triad, one study [46] tested the use of scaffold-GFs and cell-seeded scaffolds [45]. Actually, Zellner et al. [45] have compared the outcomes of PRP, hyaluronan-collagen scaffold and bone marrow as graft harvested from iliac crest of New Zealand white rabbits. The authors concluded that neither bone marrow alone nor PRP have improved healing capacity relating to acellular scaffold. However, BM-MSCs constructs performed better for healing and integration [45] as compared to all the previous.

GF's can also play a role in suture augmentation. In fact, some injuries previously considered as irreparable are now focus of attention. Kamimura et al. [50] proposed a fibrin clot approach to broaden the indication for repair of horizontal cleavage tears in the avascular zone cases. The defect was filled with fibrin clots before tightening the sutures in a "sandwich fashion". Another possibility to solve analogous problems has been reported, trying the augmentation of sutures with growth factors as VEGF [48, 49]. New approaches of bioactive agents' application for repair augmentation are subject of ongoing research [12].

9.3.2 Nanotechnology and Gene Therapy Approaches

Regenerative Medicine approaches in a broader perspective also include the use of nanotechnologies, injectable therapies and gene therapy. The latest provides the possibility of "educating" cells to produce a certain protein or reaction throughout time in a controlled matter. Nanotechnologies enable the distribution of cells, bioactive agents or drugs controlling their target or time of delivery [51], and thus allow avoiding the deleterious secondary effects of systemic drugs administration. Furthermore they all can be used combined, possibly in minimally invasive approaches or even percutaneous injections. Other nanotechnology strategies are targeted to improve the scaffolds biological performance. In a study reported by Baker et al. [52]., it was shown that electrospun aligned nanofibrous scaffolds possess a microstructural and nanoscale architecture resembling to native extracellular matrix components and provide a substrate favorable for the chondrogenic differentiation of mesenchymal stem cells.

A gene therapy approach has combined an injectable alginate gel with transfected bone marrow cells with human IGF-1 [43]. Zhang et al. [43] investigated whether bone marrow stromal cells transfected with human insulin-like growth factor 1 (hIGF-1) gene encapsulated in calcium alginate gel could improve the repair of full-thickness meniscus defects in the avascular zone of the anterior horn. Their results support the efficacy of this approach to deliver biologically effective concentrations of hIGF-1, and suggested the value of liposome-mediated ex vivo gene therapy for improving meniscus healing. Injected synovial MSCs also promoted meniscus repair without mobilization to distant organs as demonstrated by Horie et al. [53] and Mizuno et al. [54]. Agung et al. [55] reported a novel bone marrow MSCs injection approach for treating meniscal partial defects. An advanced strategy has been presented by Ochiai et al. [56], which aimed to reduce histological meniscus degeneration. Heme oxygenase-1 (HO-1) isozyme is known to mediate oxidative stress and it is negatively influenced by the Bach 1 transcription factor. In that study, it was shown an increased antioxidant activity in Bach 1 deficient mice resulting in diminished meniscus degeneration. This study opened up a new stream for research aiming to prevent osteoarthritis.

9.3.3 Conclusions–Future Trends in the Treatment of Meniscus Lesions

TERM approach enables a new vision of several old issues concerning meniscus treatment opening possibilities in the near future. It is possible to divide them academically in four issues: repair augmentation strategies; partial replacement; total meniscus replacement and prevention of joint degeneration. It is the author's belief that clinical trials involving regenerative strategies for treating meniscus lesions will be soon designed to contemplate the use of acellular "smart" and/or nanoscale-processed scaffolds, autologous cells (e.g., stem cells), bioactive agents (e.g., PRP and antibiotics). Nanotechnology is also taking part of the treatment equation as novel drug delivery systems are advantageous when the administration of drugs or antibiotics is required at lesions sites. Despite promising when cellular strategies are envisioned, gene therapy is hard to translate and thus will take longer to reach the clinical setting. This new upcoming language and area of knowledge must be understood by knee surgeons.

References

1. Verdonk R (2011) The meniscus: past, present and future. Knee Surg Sports Traumatol Arthrosc 19:145–146
2. Verdonk PC, Forsyth RG, Wang J et al (2005) Characterisation of human knee meniscus cell phenotype. Osteoarthritis Cartilage 13:548–560
3. Pereira H, Frias A, Caridade S et al (2011) Cellular and biomechanical segmental characterization of human meniscus. Osteoarthritis Cartilage 19:S205
4. Lubowitz JH, Poehling GG (2011) Save the meniscus. Arthroscopy 27:301–302
5. Elattar M, Dhollander A, Verdonk R, Almqvist KF, Verdonk P (2011) Twenty-six years of meniscal allograft transplantation: is it still experimental? A meta-analysis of 44 trials. Knee Surg Sports Traumatol Arthrosc 19:147–157 (Official journal of the ESSKA)
6. Garrett WE Jr, Swiontkowski MF, Weinstein JN et al (2006) American board of orthopaedic surgery practice of the orthopaedic surgeon: part-II, certification examination case mix. J Bone Joint Surg Am 88:660–667
7. Fayard JM, Pereira H, Servien E, Lustig S, Neyret P (2010) Meniscectomy global results-complications. Springer-Verlag, Berlin Heidelberg
8. Jackson DW (2001) The orthopaedic clinician-scientist. J Bone Joint Surg Am 83-A:131-5
9. Monllau JC, González-Lucena G, Gelber PE, Pelfort X (2010) Allograft meniscus transplantation: a current review. Tech Knee Surg 9:107–113
10. Milachowski KA, Weismeier K, Wirth CJ (1989) Homologous meniscus transplantation. Experimental and clinical results. Int Orthop 13:1–11
11. Harris JD, Cavo M, Brophy R, Siston R, Flanigan D (2011) Biological knee reconstruction: a systematic review of combined meniscal allograft transplantation and cartilage repair or restoration. Arthroscopy J Arthroscopic Relat Surg 27:409–418 (Official publication of the Arthroscopy Association of North America and the International Arthroscopy Association)
12. Pereira H, Frias AM, Oliveira JM, Espregueira-Mendes J, Reis RL (2011) Tissue engineering and regenerative medicine strategies in meniscus lesions. J Arthroscopic Related Surg 27:1706–1719 (Official publication of the Arthroscopy Association of North America and the International Arthroscopy Association)
13. Annandale T (1885) An operation for displaced semilunar cartilage. Br Med J 1:779
14. Starke C, Kopf S, Petersen W, Becker R (2009) Meniscal repair. Arthroscopy J Arthroscopic Rel Surg 25:1033–1044 (Official publication of the Arthroscopy Association of North America and the International Arthroscopy Association)
15. Logan M, Watts M, Owen J, Myers P (2009) Meniscal repair in the elite athlete: results of 45 repairs with a minimum 5-year follow-up. Am J Sports Med 37:1131–1134
16. Paxton ES, Stock MV, Brophy RH (2011) Meniscal repair versus partial meniscectomy: a systematic review comparing reoperation rates and clinical outcomes. Arthroscopy J Arthroscopic Rel Surg 27:1275–1288 (Official publication of the Arthroscopy Association of North America and the International Arthroscopy Association)
17. Muriuki MG, Tuason DA, Tucker BG, Harner CD (2011) Changes in tibiofemoral contact mechanics following radial split and vertical tears of the medial meniscus an in vitro investigation of the efficacy of arthroscopic repair. J Bone Joint Surg Am 93:1089–1095
18. Verdonk P, Beaufils P, Bellemans J et al (2012) Successful treatment of painful irreparable partial meniscal defects with a polyurethane scaffold: two-year safety and clinical outcomes. Am J Sports Med 40:844–853
19. Hirschmann MT, Keller L, Hirschmann A et al (2012) One-year clinical and MR imaging outcome after partial meniscal replacement in stabilized knees using a collagen meniscus implant. Knee Surg Sports Traumatol Arthrosc, Oct 30 2012 [Epub ahead of print]
20. Monllau JC, Gelber PE, Abat F et al (2011) Outcome after partial medial meniscus substitution with the collagen meniscal implant at a minimum of 10 years' follow-up. Arthroscopy J Arthroscopic Rel Surg 27:933–943 (Official publication of the Arthroscopy Association of North America and the International Arthroscopy Association)

21. Zaffagnini S, Marcheggiani, Muccioli GM, Lopomo N et al (2011) Prospective long-term outcomes of the medial collagen meniscus implant versus partial medial meniscectomy: a minimum 10-year follow-up study. Am J Sports Med 39(5):977–985
22. Bulgheroni P, Murena L, Ratti C, Bulgheroni E, Ronga M, Cherubino P (2010) Follow-up of collagen meniscus implant patients: clinical, radiological, and magnetic resonance imaging results at 5 years. Knee 17:224–229
23. Rodkey WG, DeHaven KE, Montgomery WH 3rd et al (2008) Comparison of the collagen meniscus implant with partial meniscectomy. A prospective randomized trial. J Bone Joint Surg Am 90:1413–1426
24. Zaffagnini S, Giordano G, Vascellari A et al (2007) Arthroscopic collagen meniscus implant results at 6–8 years follow up. Knee Surg Sports Traumatol Arthrosc 15:175–183 (Official journal of the ESSKA)
25. Linke RD, Ulmer M, Imhoff AB (2006) Replacement of the meniscus with a collagen implant (CMI). Oper Orthop Traumatol 18:453–462
26. Genovese E, Angeretti MG, Ronga M et al (2007) Follow-up of collagen meniscus implants by MRI. Radiol Med 112:1036–1048
27. Zaffagnini S, Marcheggiani, Muccioli GM, Bulgheroni P et al (2012) Arthroscopic collagen meniscus implantation for partial lateral meniscal defects: a 2-year minimum follow-up study. Am J Sports Med 40:2281–2288
28. Verdonk R, Verdonk P, Huysse W, Forsyth R, Heinrichs EL (2011) Tissue ingrowth after implantation of a novel, biodegradable polyurethane scaffold for treatment of partial meniscal lesions. Am J Sports Med 39:774–782
29. Efe T, Getgood A, Schofer MD et al (2012) The safety and short-term efficacy of a novel polyurethane meniscal scaffold for the treatment of segmental medial meniscus deficiency. Knee Surg Sports Traumatol Arthrosc 20:1822–1830 (Official journal of the ESSKA)
30. Yan LP, Oliveira JM, Oliveira AL, Caridade SG, Mano JF, Reis RL (2012) Macro/microporous silk fibroin scaffolds with potential for articular cartilage and meniscus tissue engineering applications. Acta Biomater 8:289–301
31. Kon E, Chiari C, Marcacci M et al (2008) Tissue engineering for total meniscal substitution: animal study in sheep model. Tissue Eng Part A 14:1067–1080
32. Welsing RT, van Tienen TG, Ramrattan N et al (2008) Effect on tissue differentiation and articular cartilage degradation of a polymer meniscus implant: a 2-year follow-up study in dogs. Am J Sports Med 36:1978–1989
33. Kang SW, Son SM, Lee JS et al (2006) Regeneration of whole meniscus using meniscal cells and polymer scaffolds in a rabbit total meniscectomy model. J Biomed Mater Res A 78:659–671
34. Moroni L, de Wijn JR, van Blitterswijk CA (2006) 3D fiber-deposited scaffolds for tissue engineering: Influence of pores geometry and architecture on dynamic mechanical properties. Biomaterials 27:974–985
35. Liulan L, Qingxi H, Xianxu H, Gaochun X (2007) Design and fabrication of bone tissue engineering scaffolds via rapid prototyping and CAD. J Rare Earths 25(Supplement 2):379–383
36. Angele P, Johnstone B, Kujat R et al (2008) Stem cell based tissue engineering for meniscus repair. J Biomed Mater Res A 85:445–455
37. Scotti C, Pozzi A, Mangiavini L et al (2009) Healing of meniscal tissue by cellular fibrin glue: an in vivo study. Knee Surg Sports Traumatol Arthrosc 17:645–651
38. Weinand C, Xu JW, Peretti GM, Bonassar LJ, Gill TJ (2009) Conditions affecting cell seeding onto three-dimensional scaffolds for cellular-based biodegradable implants. J Biomed Mater Res B Appl Biomater 91:80–87
39. Yamasaki T, Deie M, Shinomiya R, Yasunaga Y, Yanada S, Ochi M (2008) Transplantation of meniscus regenerated by tissue engineering with a scaffold derived from a rat meniscus and mesenchymal stromal cells derived from rat bone marrow. Artif Organs 32:519–524

40. Martinek V, Ueblacker P, Braun K et al (2006) Second generation of meniscus transplantation: in vivo study with tissue engineered meniscus replacement. Arch Orthop Trauma Surg 126:228–234
41. Weinand C, Peretti GM, Adams SB Jr, Bonassar LJ, Randolph MA, Gill TJ (2006) An allogenic cell-based implant for meniscal lesions. Am J Sports Med 34:1779–1789
42. Weinand C, Peretti GM, Adams SB Jr, Randolph MA, Savvidis E, Gill TJ (2006) Healing potential of transplanted allogeneic chondrocytes of three different sources in lesions of the avascular zone of the meniscus: a pilot study. Arch Orthop Trauma Surg 126:599–605
43. Zhang H, Leng P, Zhang J (2009) Enhanced meniscal repair by overexpression of hIGF-1 in a full-thickness model. Clin Orthop Relat Res 467:3165–3174
44. Kobayashi Y, Yasuda K, Kondo E et al (2010) Implantation of autogenous meniscal fragments wrapped with a fascia sheath enhances fibrocartilage regeneration in vivo in a large harvest site defect. Am J Sports Med 38:740–748
45. Zellner J, Mueller M, Berner A et al (2010) Role of mesenchymal stem cells in tissue engineering of meniscus. J Biomed Mater Res A 94:1150–1161
46. Stapleton TW, Ingram J, Fisher J, Ingham E (2011) Investigation of the regenerative capacity of an acellular porcine medial meniscus for tissue engineering applications. Tissue Eng Part A 17:231–242
47. Ishida K, Kuroda R, Miwa M et al (2007) The regenerative effects of platelet-rich plasma on meniscal cells in vitro and its in vivo application with biodegradable gelatin hydrogel. Tissue Eng 13:1103–1112
48. Kopf S, Birkenfeld F, Becker R et al (2010) Local treatment of meniscal lesions with vascular endothelial growth factor. J Bone Joint Surg Am 92:2682–2691
49. Petersen W, Pufe T, Starke C et al (2007) The effect of locally applied vascular endothelial growth factor on meniscus healing: gross and histological findings. Arch Orthop Trauma Surg 127:235–240
50. Kamimura T, Kimura M (2011) Repair of horizontal meniscal cleavage tears with exogenous fibrin clots. Knee Surg Sports Traumatol Arthrosc 19(7):1154–1157
51. Abdel-Mohsen AM, Hrdina R, Burgert L et al (2012) Antibacterial activity and cell viability of hyaluronan fiber with silver nanoparticles. Carbohydrate Polymers 92:1177–1187
52. Baker BM, Nathan AS, Gee AO, Mauck RL (2010) The influence of an aligned nanofibrous topography on human mesenchymal stem cell fibrochondrogenesis. Biomaterials 31:6190–6200
53. Horie M, Sekiya I, Muneta T et al (2009) Intra-articular Injected synovial stem cells differentiate into meniscal cells directly and promote meniscal regeneration without mobilization to distant organs in rat massive meniscal defect. Stem Cells 27:878–887
54. Mizuno K, Muneta T, Morito T et al (2008) Exogenous synovial stem cells adhere to defect of meniscus and differentiate into cartilage cells. J Med Dent Sci 55:101–111
55. Agung M, Ochi M, Yanada S et al (2006) Mobilization of bone marrow-derived mesenchymal stem cells into the injured tissues after intraarticular injection and their contribution to tissue regeneration. Knee Surg Sports Traumatol Arthrosc 14:1307–1314
56. Ochiai S, Mizuno T, Deie M, Igarashi K, Hamada Y, Ochi M (2008) Oxidative stress reaction in the meniscus of bach 1 deficient mice: potential prevention of meniscal degeneration. J Orthop Res 26:894–898

Part IV
Conclusion

Conclusion

10

R. Verdonk, J. C. Monllau and J. Espregueira-Mendes

Now that everything has been said about the meniscus, we have to come to a conclusion regarding the issues still facing us.

Meniscal diagnosis has come a long way. Clinical examination and patient history have been supplemented with other diagnostic tools such as digital-precision imaging. It still remains the orthopaedic surgeon's prerogative to take into account any of these and to tailor the treatment to the individual patient, while relating the clinical information to his experience.

On the other hand, imaging is black-and-white information—soon maybe more colourful—and needs to be put into perspective, taking into account the patient's complaints and physical limitations. Therefore, the combination of both worlds is essential, but may sometimes be difficult, even for the seasoned orthopaedic surgeon.

Once designated as the "gold standard" for the diagnosis of meniscus pathology, arthroscopy has currently become part of the therapeutic arsenal, because effective treatment can be associated to this type of surgery. It is now realized that even at that stage a common denomination of the same pathology remains difficult.

R. Verdonk (✉)
Dept Orthopaedics and Trauma, University Hospital, De Pintelaan 185, 9000 Ghent, Belgium
e-mail: Rene.verdonk@ugent.be

J. C. Monllau
Department of Orthopaedic Surgery, Hospital de la Sta Creu i Sant Pau, ICATME–Institut Universitari Dexeus, Universitat Autònoma de Barcelona., St AM Claret, 167, 08025 Barcelona, Spain
e-mail: Jmonllau@santpau.cat

J. Espregueira-Mendes
Clínica Espregueira-Mendes, Estádio do Dragão, 4350-415 Porto, Portugal
e-mail: jem@espregueira.com

R. Verdonk et al. (eds.), *Meniscal Transplantation*,
DOI: 10.1007/978-3-642-38106-5_10, © ISAKOS 2013

Only recently Committees (ISAKOS—Allan Anderson) have come to a conclusion on common denomination of the pathology at hand.

In fact, the steps towards confronting the tentative preoperative diagnosis with the actual findings are being taken every day in orthopaedic diagnosis.

Arthroscopy has paved the way for straightforward arthroscopic surgery of the menisci. The concept of these being "vestigial" structures (Scott Dye) has long been refuted. The integrity of these semilunar cartilages is respected more and more as they are handled with care.

Because adequate resection has become the standard of care whenever appropriate, surgery and suture of the meniscus have gained importance in the armamentarium of surgical procedures.

With this has come an explosion of devices designed to obtain satisfactory stabilization of the torn part(s), which leads to good long-term clinical results. The relation of the torn meniscus to other traumatic lesions inside the knee—ACL, PCL, collateral ligaments—has sustained the importance of combined lesions and their treatment over time.

Long-term results have clearly shown the importance of both healed menisci and stable ligament structures to the cartilage surface of the knee, this being a prerequisite for the long-term integrity of this weight bearing joint.

However, once a treatment has led to adequate and sometimes dramatic resection, the "slippery slope" (Peter Verdonk) concept comes into play. Most often, combined resection of the meniscus and loss of ligament balance will require proper treatment.

Tissue loss requires replacement as does loss of stability. Ligament replacement has proven to be the standard of care. Meniscal replacement is still an ongoing field of research.

When confronted with total resection, total replacement with allografts has proven to be a valuable alternative with satisfactory long-term outcomes. Deep-frozen, cryopreserved, and viable allografts tend to provide 70 % of near-satisfactory results whatever the preservation technique used. This is particularly true for the lateral compartment of the knee.

However, the number of these cases is limited, because most often only partial meniscectomy has been performed with preservation of the meniscal wall. This has led the way to partial replacement of the meniscus, exploring new concepts of implants capable of withstanding physiological stress, strain and loads in the knee joint.

In this emerging field of clinical science, research has led to the development of fascinating new products, such as the collagen meniscus implant (Steadman—Rodkey) and a polyurethane scaffold (Jacqueline De Groot) designed to recreate normal homeostasis and thus a painfree and hopefully long-lasting, well-functioning knee.

Thus, researchers and clinicians are trying to beat the odds by searching for a replacement structure, resorbable yet strong enough to allow time for ingrowth of the "meniscal" cell so as to replace the implant scaffold with new-woven own collagen. This cell, the typing of which is still not fully understood, partly originates from the vascularized synovium but also from the knee joint itself, as provider of a stimulating medium.

Today's knowledge of knee meniscus physiology and pathology, as presented by the renowned authors in this work, might be a stimulus for a future breakthrough.

MIX
Papier aus verantwortungsvollen Quellen
Paper from responsible sources
FSC® C105338

If you have any concerns about our products,
you can contact us on
ProductSafety@springernature.com

In case Publisher is established outside the EU,
the EU authorized representative is:
Springer Nature Customer Service Center GmbH
Europaplatz 3, 69115 Heidelberg, Germany

Printed by Libri Plureos GmbH
in Hamburg, Germany